QUIET PLEASE

QUIET PLEASE

Tinnitus and My Journey through Self-Discovery

SEAN WEATHERILL

ISBN: 978-1-09-469858-8

Interior book design by *the*BookDesigners

Printed in the United States of America

For Catlin with all my gratitude and love

PREFACE

This book is about a journey that started with my diagnosis of tinnitus but ended with so much more. If you had told me three years ago that tinnitus was here to help me, I would have told you to go fuck yourself. Today, I'm not so sure. It seems that tinnitus has caused far more good in my life than bad, and while mine has been a painful—and sometimes excruciating—learning process, it has also been a necessary one. In fact, my journey has taken me to places I never would have gone without the noise in my head. What began as an obsession to find a cure transformed into a deeply personal journey encompassing health, fitness, love, learning, and spirituality. This is the story of my journey.

January 2018

I am back in the house for the third time, lying on the floor on what feels like a bed of pillows. There's a mask over my eyes. Tears stream down my face. Every few minutes, I take huge deep breaths in and out. For the most part, though, I am oblivious to the outside world. My focus is turned inward, to where my Self is being led up a tube by a very sweet and small fairy spirit. Holding tightly to my right hand, she takes me to places that lie deep within my soul and even deeper within my unconscious. She reveals to me everything my heart has always known about spirituality but has not yet been shown.

"Come on, I have lots of things I want to show you," she says.

"What about my tinnitus?" I reply. "Isn't that why I'm here?"

"You seem to be doing pretty well with that," she notes. "Now come on, let's go."

And we do. Before long, I feel a hand on my chest and lots of pressure. It's my mom's hand—my mom who had passed away just two months before. She tells me that it's going to be okay, that she's still with me, that she will always be with me, and that she is sorry for leaving. The tears pour from my eyes as I feel a cathartic release of pain and sadness. Then, almost as quickly as she appeared, she vanishes again into time and space. I'm a young boy again—seven years old—and I can see my dad standing not too far away. I don't run to him. My spirit guide speaks up from my side.

"Did you ever receive any love from your father?" she asks.

"No," I reply quickly. "None at all."

"And how did that feel?"

"It hurt a lot," I said. "It still hurts."

"Without this love, how did you become such a loving person and father?"

"I got it from my mom," I reply, "and from my wife, Catlin."

A few minutes later, or perhaps a few hours, it's hard to tell, I'm once again in a different place. This time, it's my childhood bedroom. I'm a young boy on the top bunk of my bed, scared to death, as a huge, mad dog paces around on the floor below, snarling and barking at me. He comes to my room often, trapping me on my bed. It's always the same story. He's terrifying, but he never wakes my older brother who is lying on the bunk below. It seems he is only after me. After what feels like hours, I summon the courage to jump off the bed and make a run for it. The mad dog is on my heels, snapping at me. As quickly as I can, I escape into my mom's room, where she comforts me. My dad is there, too, but I receive no comfort from him. The fear subsides for a moment. Then I feel fearful again. I am still a young boy, and I'm having a nightmare. It's the one I have had many times before, the one that makes me scared to close my eyes at night. I wake up, terrified, and run to the bathroom to vomit. I cannot recall the nightmare; I just know that it was tremendously awful. My mom is there comforting me, like always, filled with love. I try to engage my guide again.

"But what about my tinnitus?" I reiterate.

"Oh Sean," she sighs, "Always trying to control everything. Come on, I have so much more to show you."

Five hours later, I am out of the mask. I feel like I have been ripped apart from the inside out and reassembled into what will eventually become a better version of myself. I look different and almost unrecognizable. My face is red and puffy. Dried tears cover my neck. Somehow, I also look energized. There is a glow to me, like switches have been turned on for the first time in forty years. I struggle to put into words what I have experienced. Brutal, powerful, wonderful, terrifying. One thing I know for sure, though, is that tinnitus or no tinnitus, I am never, ever going back into that space again. I'm not sure I could survive it a second time. Yet, as I leave the house, I pause to consider everything that has brought me to this moment and am amazed by what I have gone through and how much I have already overcome.

When I arrive home, Catlin is there to greet me. "How was it, love? What did you learn?"

"Everything," I say. "I learned everything."

INTRODUCTION

TINNITUS: A medical condition that causes ringing or roaring sounds that only you can hear.

I have had tinnitus, or T as I'll call it, for about four years now and they have been, without a doubt, the most difficult four years of my life. It's remarkable how something so mysterious, secret, and internal can be so disruptive. My journey with T has been exhausting, sometimes overwhelming, and occasionally debilitating. Even as I write this, it is here with me—it is always here—but it doesn't drive me crazy like it used to. Sometimes I wonder if I'll come to a point where I'll be glad to have T around. Or maybe it will disappear from my life altogether. No matter my personal outcome, through my journey, I have discovered another side to T and have been able to embrace the lessons that have come from having it. While every individual's experience with T is different, my hope is that by sharing my story, I might help others living with T, especially those suffering silently.

When my symptoms first appeared, I was told by both my primary care doctor at Kaiser Permanente and by a private doctor in San Francisco that my T was the result of mid-range hearing loss. That explanation didn't sit right with me. Something inside me knew there was more to the story. Sure, I might have some mild or even moderate mid-range hearing loss, but I was not at all convinced that it was the cause of the ringing in my head. Instead, I intuited that it indicated something much deeper; I saw it as a tea kettle going off, a warning sign that the heat needed to be turned down in some part of my life or that the pressure was far too high. Was I under too much stress? Was I working too much? Was I holding on to something I shouldn't? Did I have a bunch of old shit buried deep in my unconscious? I knew the answer to all of these questions was yes, and I felt strongly that my psyche was the driving force behind my T, rather than my inner-ear condition. The experts were telling me that I was wrong, but they seemed to be trying to just shuffle me along, perhaps in order to move on to their next patient.

I quickly learned that T can turn your life upside down. It can ruin your days and fill your nights with nightmares. Seeking help can backfire; the more you research, the more people with whom you consult, the more scared and hopeless you can become.

For anyone out there currently struggling with T, I know how awful it can be. Hang in there. It can get better. Even if the sound never leaves you, your experience of it can change dramatically. I know because I've changed my own experience of my own T. I am writing this book because I want to help you cope and, perhaps, to help you conquer your tinnitus altogether.

My personal journey has not been easy, but the outcome has been well worth the grueling work. When I decided to reclaim my life from T, I was forced to try new things, to work on self-discipline, and to take major leaps of faith. What I didn't know going into my process was that it would be my journey itself that would lead me to the results I wanted.

I do not claim to be a doctor or expert in the field of T. This is simply the story of my journey and my personal experiences. Naturally, it contains my own opinions.

Meet Mr. T

One more quick note. I started writing this book using the condition's full name 'tinnitus,' but I hate that word and hated looking at it, not because of what it is, but just because I think the word is ugly. So I switched to using T for much of this book. However, during my journey, I began to understand 'My T' better, which is when Mr. T came onto the scene. Mr. T is my own private version of T; you will come to know him well, too, as you read on.

CHAPTER 1

THE SET-UP

One day, a few years ago, I was at my parents' house and saw an ad on TV for a prescription drug claiming to help people suffering from something called tinnitus. I had never heard of it before. The ad showed adults in their 60s and 70s holding their hands over their ears to try to stop the noise. I remember thinking, "Wow, that sounds awful," before continuing on with my day.

A couple of months later, at the age of 46, I was on an annual mountain-biking trip with a bunch of friends. Early one morning, I was lying in my tent when I noticed a slight, high-pitched noise in my right ear. "That's curious," I thought. "I wonder if I need to get my ears cleaned." I didn't focus much on the noise at the time, but I certainly noticed it every morning and every evening for several months. The sound was always there, or at least when I caught myself thinking about it. And I was starting to think about it more and more.

Bad Ideas

After a few months of living with the sound in my ear, I decided to do some research on the internet to see what I could learn about what was going on. Of course, this was a terrible idea. I'm quite sure I'm not the only person with undiagnosed tinnitus who has searched

Google with some version of "ringing in my ear," only to have the crap scared out of them. The more I read, the more I felt the need to deny that I might be suffering from this awful condition. "This can't be me, can it? I'm too young, too healthy, and, and, and…"

I was worried. Very worried. While I still hoped that the noise would go away on its own, the seeds of fear had been planted and were preparing to sprout and grow like weeds in my mind. Fear was a powerful fertilizer; my awareness of the ringing was heightened, and there was no going back. I started to constantly track the noise. The more I researched, the more scared and obsessed with the noise I became. I was aware that I had given this monster wings, and it was going to fly far and high.

Eventually, I decided to make an appointment with a physician to get my ears checked. At the time, I was a member of Kaiser Permanente. While Kaiser continues to be a great option for my wife and kids, my particular doctor didn't work for me. At my appointment, I explained to him what was going on with the noise in my ears. After a few minutes of exchanging pleasantries, he looked in my ears and said, "You probably have T. If it doesn't go away in a couple of months, you will likely have it forever."

"Wait," I thought, "Forever? Surely, there must be a way for me to fix this. What should I do?"

I was panicked, scared, and seeking reassurance. The doctor simply told me to come back in a couple of months and sent me on my way, still absolutely terrified. Subsequently, my obsession with my T grew. My focus on the noise increased over time, which made it exponentially worse. It started to affect my ability to sleep at night and my capacity to function during the day. My days were consumed by that fucking ringing in my ears.

One of my general life coping mechanisms and stress-relievers at the time was working out at the gym with friends. About six months into my life with T, one of my coaches at the gym, who also happens to be a great friend, asked me how I was doing.

"Not great," I told her. "I have tinnitus and it's been really hard for me to to deal with."

Trying to sympathize, she said, "Oh man, that sucks, Sean. I've heard that can drive people crazy! I mean, that's why Van Gogh cut his ear off, isn't it?"

No doubt, her intention was to comfort me and let me know she understood the severity of my condition. She wasn't trying to scare me. She had no idea how terrified and vulnerable I was, and her comment only served to exacerbate my fears.

I started to feel like every time I reached out for support, I got kicked in the nuts instead.

The Break

About eight months into my life with Mr. T., I was at a good friend's house with my wife, Catlin, and another close friend. We were hanging out in the hot tub. The jets were going, and they were super loud, but the ringing in my ear was louder still. "How can it be," I wondered, "that I'm in a hot tub, with people talking and jets roaring, and all I can hear is my T?"

I decided to have a drink or two to drown out the ringing. Unfortunately, it made matters worse. I ended up having a breakdown of sorts, or maybe it could be described as a panic attack. My friend offered me a Valium. I took it and, after an hour or so, I calmed down.

I had been suffering mostly silently for eight months prior to that night in the hot tub, so nobody had really known what was going on with me. Of course, Catlin knew I had been struggling with my T, but I don't think she knew the full extent of the problem. My other two friends had known nothing. What transpired around the hot tub wasn't exactly how I'd imagined letting my friends in on my big secret. But it was becoming increasingly clear that I was not in control of the T situation. In fact, it felt like I was no longer in control of much anymore.

I couldn't help but wonder, "Is this how my life is going to be from now on?"

Deep down, I knew this was just the beginning of what would be a long and arduous journey. It was possible the noise would stay the same, but I also knew it could get even worse.

As it turned out, the breakdown by the hot tub would set the stage for how I would manage my T for the next year. I would do whatever I could to avoid the ringing, especially at night. My M.O. every day involved two to four drinks after 5:00, half (or more) of a 10 mg Valium, and then some wine. Sometimes I also indulged in a night cap of Nyquil. This was the best way I knew how to cope, and, as you might imagine, it wasn't very effective.

A Few More Bad Ideas

After living for some months in my own private hell, I decided to return to my doctor at Kaiser. I told him I couldn't sleep, and he offered me some Ambien and a heavy prescription of Prednisone. I had taken Prednisone in the past for a bad case of bronchitis, so I knew it wouldn't work for me. I tried the sleeping pills, but they just spun me out even more.

I truly believe that going to this doctor was one of the biggest mistakes I could have made in relation to my desire to get well. He instilled fear and hopelessness. After my second visit, I felt very much alone and couldn't sleep at all. I was scared to talk to anyone about my T because it seemed like every time I did, it made things worse.

A while later, I chose to see a different doctor, this time an ear specialist outside of my network, in the hopes of getting some good news. She was the first person to do a hearing test on me, and she was pleasant and nice, a welcome contrast to Dr. Frankenstein over at Kaiser.

But when she returned with the results, she said, "Well, you have some mid-range hearing loss, and that's probably what's causing the ringing in your ear. It may get worse. It probably won't get better. There are some ways you can try to cope with it, but there's not much you can do to fix it altogether."

"Why did I even come here, then?" I thought.

A Spark of Hope
Mixed With a Lot of Fear

Shortly thereafter, while visiting one of my work sites—I'm a landscape designer and contractor—I was so on edge that I could barely focus. I could tell that I was on the verge of another breakdown when my phone rang. It was my good friend, Steve, calling from San Diego to check in on me. It was like he somehow knew that I needed help right then and there. Already very emotional from a challenging morning, I could barely keep it together on the phone. Steve did most of the talking, while I quietly got my shit together. Our conversation went something like this:

Steve- Hey, I just wanted to check in and see how you're doing.

Sean- Not great, actually.

Steve- What's up?

Sean- I have this ringing in my ears.

Steve- Oh, you mean tinnitus?

Sean- Yes.

Steve- I have that, too. I've had it for about ten years now.

I felt a huge wave of relief and hope sweep over me. Steve was the first person I knew to also suffer from T. He told me that he had learned to manage it and that it had never worsened. He had gotten it at around the same age as me, and he was now 54 and doing great.

Then the conversation shifted. Steve told me about some of his friends who also had tinnitus, but who had more extreme cases than he did. A few of them, he said, had to wear earphones because the sound was as loud as a train.

"Now," he said, "that's when you put the 45 in your mouth."

"Here we go again." Just like that, my first hopeful, positive conversation about T had presented me with my deepest fear. I couldn't handle the idea that T might drive me completely mad.

I just kept thinking, "Why? Why me?" Everything else was pretty great in my life. I had the most wonderful partner in the world, two great kids, and a pretty loving family. I was healthy, or at least I thought I was, and very active. Why was my world being turned upside-down by this high-pitched noise?

The Spiral Down

By that point, my days and nights were consumed with trying to drown out the noise. Was it getting worse? Was it on my left side now, too? Was I going crazy? I would drive on the freeway at 80 MPH with the windows down, but all I could hear was that fucking high-pitched noise, whirring like a hard drive on a computer. I was consumed with the thought that it was going to get worse and then I wouldn't be able to handle it anymore.

At night, I would lie in bed with the windows open to see if I could distinguish between the crickets out back and my T. Then, I would climb into the shower, as that was the only way I could escape the sound. Catlin would often find me there at 3:00 am.

"Love, are you okay?" she would ask.

"Yes," I would reply. "I'm just trying to get a break from the noise."

But I was far from OK. I was exhausted, scared, and desperate.

I was frantic to find something that would fix my problem. Still not convinced that it was mid-range hearing loss causing my T, I decided to explore all of the other possible explanations. Was it from too much caffeine? Too much alcohol? Too much stress or too much salt? Too much exercise or too much gluten? Was it neck problems? What about work problems?

I was operating in panic mode. Alcohol and Valium fueled my functioning. I felt like I was drowning alone, with no help or solution in sight. My fear was at a level ten. My focus was completely on Mr. T, and I dreaded both going to bed and waking up. I was in a dark place. My one saving grace was my wife and kids. No matter how scared I got, I knew that I had to push on and find a solution, or at least some relief, so that I could get back to our great life together.

Down and Out

While researching, I learned that some people with T had found success and relief from chiropractic adjustments, and I wondered if they could help me, too. Since my good friend Tyler has a chiropractic/sports therapy practice in San Diego, I booked a flight and headed down to meet him. I hadn't told him about my T yet. He just thought I was coming in to get worked on for another CrossFit injury. He worked on me for about an hour, doing the usual, painful treatment, which had me stretching and twisting and writhing around, all in the name of healing. When we were done, I mentioned T.

"Oh man," he said, "you know how serious that can be, right? I had a friend who had it and jumped off the Golden Gate Bridge."

"Fucking great. Thanks, Tyler," I thought.

At the time, I lived a short ten miles from the Golden Gate Bridge.

Tyler is a great guy. He wasn't trying to scare me, but, like my gym coach, he just didn't realize how freaked out and vulnerable I already was. Afterwards, he looked at my neck again and said that he was pretty sure my T was caused by something mechanical, rather than by hearing loss. Because it was a new explanation with a possible road to treatment, it actually gave me some hope.

Still, it felt like every time I tried something new, and every time I talked to someone about my T for the first time, I was left with fear and disappointment. Although I had no plans of ending my search for relief,

I wasn't feeling very hopeful overall. I was already more than a year into my dance with the terror that is Mr. T, and I was a mess.

Of course, there were moments throughout the day when I was focused on something else and didn't notice Mr. T, but those moments were becoming fewer and further between. I was obsessed with my condition. I constantly monitored it. I would stick my fingers in my ears to see where it was coming from and how loud it was.

I don't know how best to describe it to someone who does not have T, but for me it's a constant high pitch whistle coming from both sides. It fluctuates throughout the day and night, sometimes up, sometimes down, but never fully quiet. Have you ever been to a concert or had something happen that left your ears ringing for a few hours? Having T is like that, but it never goes away. Instead, it's constantly tapping on my shoulder, making sure I don't forget about it or ignore it. The reminders are relentless. If Mr. T could talk, I feel like he might say any one of the following, at any given moment:

-"Hey, don't you forget about me, not even for a second!"

-"How about a little higher on the left?"

-"How about I drive up the pitch?"

-"How about I wake you up in the middle of the night and scare the shit out of you?"

-"How about I make you think that I am going to get way louder in the coming years?"

-"Oh, you're trying to drown me out with some other sound? How cute. Good luck with that, fucker;

I'm way deeper than any external noise, and nothing can stop me."

My particular frequency is very high, or maybe I would call it bright and sharp. It's not a buzz like a high-voltage line, but more like the highest pitch a cricket could make, resounding constantly and repeatedly in my ears.

As a result, I usually don't need to be reminded that my T is there, because it's just so torturous and annoying that I am usually tracking it, no matter what else is going on. Best case scenario, I may get totally engaged in something and let it slip from my mind for a brief time, but Mr. T is like a panther. He doesn't let me go for long, and he pounces at the first opportunity. I may be free for a few minutes or even an hour, but when I give him even a millisecond of space, he jabs his claws into me again.

He also totally ruins my focus. Even while deep in conversation with someone or doing something like writing this book, a part of me is aware of Mr. T and watching him. It feels as though I've had to develop two separate minds: one that allows me to function like a normal human being, and another that tracks that fucking panther. If I am lucky, I will get into some sort of flow state, and the panther will drop behind. But then there are other times when the panther is on top of me, flashing its claws and tearing at me, paralyzing me and preventing me from doing anything else. I just sit there, afraid.

CHAPTER 2

THE NEED FOR CHANGE

CrossFit or Not-Fit?

I first started doing CrossFit in 2010, prior to T entering my life, and was immediately hooked. There was a new "box" not far from where I lived, and, after several months of thinking about going in, I finally did. There, I met Marcus, one of the gym's owners. Marcus was super fit and a bit intimidating at first, but he was also a committed athlete and coach. We became friends, and his athleticism inspired me. He helped me learn the ropes so that, after spending a few long months in the introductory course, I felt ready to step into group classes. Ultimately, I discovered much more at that gym than just a workout; I found a whole new world filled with people who would become my closest friends.

After T came on the scene, I started working out even more, since my CrossFit class seemed to offer me some relief. It was loud, and when it was time to do the workout, I focused on that instead of the internal noise. The problem was that my T always seemed to get worse after class. I concluded that this must be due to the increased blood flow in and around my ears (my own professional, medical opinion, of course). I was okay with this possibility, because it seemed to support my theory that my T wasn't caused by my hearing after all. I mean, if I could increase the noise, then surely I should be able to find a way to decrease it, right? I became a CrossFit machine, working out every day, often twice a day, riding the high and the buzz, and putting myself to sleep each night with a mixture of alcohol, Valium, and Nyquil. I wondered if I'd ever experience peace and quiet again.

For a time, Marcus became my personal coach at the gym, which meant that he asked me lots of questions, not only about workouts, but also about lifestyle, sleeping, and eating. When it was time for our first sit-down, I told Marcus about my struggles with Mr. T.

He replied, "Oh man, Sean, that really sucks, but I know you can get through it. That shit isn't normal. It's not normal to have ringing in your ears all the time. I think you need to make a whole bunch of changes."

He recommended significant changes to my diet and lifestyle. Although he had a lot of it right, I wasn't in a good enough place in my head to take full advantage of his advice at the time. Looking back, many of his suggestions, including meditation, breathing exercises, stretching, better sleep habits, and healthier eating, are key parts of my regimen today.

Ironically, to most of the people in my gym community, I seemed to be doing great. I certainly appeared to be in good shape, but nobody knew about the internal battle I was fighting with Mr. T. On the outside, I was fit, but on the inside, I wasn't fit at all. I actually felt totally out of control and uncontained.

I would often force myself to go to the gym in the morning, just so I could try to clean out my system from the poisons of the night before. I began to see that if I ever wanted to be myself again, I would have to make some significant changes. I would need to somehow become far more mentally strong than I was at the time. Of course, this was just a thought. I had no plan yet, nor was I equipped to execute any changes, but something inside me told me this would be the only way to beat my T.

Just Breathe, then Freeze, Part I

In early 2016, two years into my new life, I was listening to a Joe Rogan Experience podcast when Wim Hof came on to discuss his breathing exercises and the Wim Hof Method (WHM). He said it could help with a litany of problems. Although he didn't mention T specifically, I was desperate and figured I should give it a try.

That night, I purchased his online course and started the breathing exercises. I actually found them very challenging, and they seemed to make my T worse. I quit after about a week.

The second part of the WHM involved cold showers. I absolutely hate cold water and being cold in general, so the idea of taking a cold shower sounded awful to me.

"But what the hell?" I thought. "I have to try. Maybe it's the key to getting my life back on track."

So I did as Hof suggested in his video course. It was winter in Northern California at the time, and the tap water was pretty damn cold. I found it hard to force my hand to turn the dial, but I managed to do it. The water came out, and I briefly stepped into its arctic blast.

"Okay," I thought, "round one done. Now can you do 30 more seconds? What about a minute? What about five?"

I noticed two things the cold water had done right away. One, it had made me forget about my T and, for that matter, everything else. Two, it had made me feel good, at least afterwards.

I tried to keep at it for a few weeks, but it was definitely a love-hate relationship, which meant that I only did it when I was feeling especially desperate and tortured. My trial with the WHM came to an end fairly soon after it had begun…at least for a while.

MTB Trip Gone Wrong
May 2016

For the past 30 years, I have been a pretty avid mountain bike rider. It's always been my escape, a way to clear my head, and I generally feel great after a ride. But after T struck, things were different. I couldn't drown out the constant noise with a good ride. Instead, my internal monologue on the topic went something like this: "Okay, I'll just ride with earbuds in…Crap, I have my music turned almost all the way up and that fucking noise is still there." And the louder I had to turn up the music, the more freaked out I became. I tried my best to get out there and ride, but everything had changed, and now what was once my sanctuary felt more like a living hell.

I have a group of friends with whom I have ridden for more than 20 years. Occasionally, we go on an international biking trip. For many years, I would go on a trip about once every four years. In the Winter of 2015, the group invited me to ride with them in Italy, a trip they were planning for the late Spring of 2016. It sounded amazing--mountain biking, the Dolomites, and cappuccinos and beers after riding through medieval towns.

Physically, I was not ready for the trip. Skill-wise, I was not ready for the trip. Mentally, I was not ready for the trip. But I thought it might be good for me, so I told them to sign me up.

When the time came, I packed everything I needed, including some Valium and Nyquil, and headed for the airport. Although I wanted the insurance, I was pretty convinced I wouldn't need the sleep and life-coping aides. I mean, I was going to be riding in Italy. I figured my mind would need to be so focused on surviving deadly exposure and hugging the trail on the edge of cliffs at 25 MPH that it wouldn't be possible for me to even tune in to my T. When I wasn't on the bike, I would be eating amazing food like gelato and touring ancient ruins. How could the noise in my head compete with that?

On the third day of riding, we were high up in the mountains in the middle of fucking nowhere. My riding had been off. My head wasn't in the game, and I knew that if I didn't get my shit together soon, I would end up making a mistake and falling off a cliff. Honestly, I didn't want to be there. I wanted to be back home with Catlin and the kids, where I had a better shot at managing things like my T.

It had been driving me crazy on the trail. I couldn't get away from it. I'm all for having a riding partner, but "Mr. T" was causing me nothing but problems and not offering anything in return. Meanwhile, I was riding so much more slowly than everyone else that I had been left in the dust. I started feeling like I was going to have a breakdown or a panic attack, right there in the middle of the Dolomites, all alone.

"Holy crap," I thought, "this is not good." I pulled over and stuck my fingers in my ears to try to get a read on things. It was the same old sound, nothing worse than normal, so why panic?

Looking back, I think the biggest problem was that I had left the place where I had learned to manage Mr. T to some extent. At home, I had a routine in place and escape routes planned for when I needed them. I had support from Catlin, and I had my kids. They could always lighten the load when I needed to feel better. In Italy, I was on my own, and I was not prepared for it. I had thought that having Valium on hand would be enough, but clearly I had underestimated just how fucked up I really was.

As I stood there on the trail next to my bike, I tried to decide how this was all going to go down. As I saw it, I had three options. One: I could have a breakdown right then and there and would be forced to let everyone in on my little secret. I'd have to let them all know that I had a roommate named Mr. T who lived in my head and was driving me crazy. Two: I could try to pull myself together by taking some Valium and hope that it didn't make my riding worse. Three: I could ride on, and hope for the best. I opted for the Valium, got back on the bike, and, about 30-45 minutes later, I felt calmer. I still wasn't riding well, but at least I was no longer anticipating a breakdown.

That night, after a few beers, some wine, half a Valium, and some Nyquil, I slept like shit. Go figure. If Mr. T wanted to ruin my trip, he was doing a damn good job of it. Almost every night, I had to put in ear-buds and listen to Kid Rock just so I could relax. Sleep was out of the question.

Ultimately, I survived the trip, but I was ecstatic when it was time to board the plane and head home.

The whole thing proved to be a wake-up call of sorts. It showed me how screwed up I was and how serious things were. I learned that, stripped of the various protections I had built up over the previous three years, I was super vulnerable. Unfortunately, when I returned, I still didn't have a plan to get well. While I was exploring options, my coping mechanisms consisted mostly of Valium and alcohol. But I promised myself I would never go on another international mountain biking trip again. It was just too hard.

I felt isolated and alone and was so afraid to talk to anyone about my condition. I was paralyzed by the fear that they would either tell me some horror story or discount what I was going through by saying it was all in my head. Both had happened one too many times already. That latter response especially infuriates me to this day.

Headspace This

Of course, I knew that I needed to stop relying so much on the alcohol and Valium. I'm a rational, otherwise highly functioning person and didn't doubt that something needed to change. "Maybe if I can calm my mind," I thought, "I can calm down Mr. T, too."

And so, in the fall of 2016, I decided to give meditation a try. I knew going into it that quieting everything would be close to impossible for me. After all, I couldn't even quiet my mind for a second. How would I ever be able to achieve a state of nirvana? But I knew I had to try.

I researched mobile meditation apps, found *Headspace*, and immediately downloaded it and started the ten-day introduction. The first sessions lasted for only minutes, and I did them every day, just like the app recommended.

After I finished the introduction, I decided to sign up for the monthly membership, so I could keep working at it. Unfortunately, I never experienced anything even remotely close to what I would call meditation, and certainly not nirvana. In fact, it often felt like the complete opposite. Since most of the time with the app was pretty quiet, it was usually just me and Mr. T sitting there fuming at one another. I suffered through, hoping for some kind of breakthrough, but it never came.

I liked the idea of *Headspace*, and I thought the coaching and the app as a whole were exceptional, but sitting there trying to have a clear mind while Mr. T was riding my ass proved impossible for me. It's possible that I didn't give the app a fair chance (I only used it about 30 times altogether), but I felt that if I was going to learn to meditate, I would have to do it another way. So I took a break from meditation, but that introduction did teach me some valuable lessons that I would find useful later down the road.

Dread the Bed

Prior to the emergence of Mr. T in my life, I always loved going to bed. Mr. T changed all that. I started dreading bedtime. I no longer slept with Catlin. Instead, I would usually find my way to one of the vacant kids' rooms to lie down and suffer alone. I tried fans, sound apps, earbuds, anything. Nothing helped. My best bet was to get enough tequila or wine in me, mix it with Valium when necessary, fall asleep watching TV, and then rouse myself just enough to stumble my way into a bed. Even still, I would wake up many times throughout the night, tossing and turning, and eventually I'd end up in the shower with a glass of wine at 3:00 am. The shower was truly the only place where I could escape the noise. As soon as I shut off the water, Mr. T was back.

Every night was filled with fear and despair. It felt like there was a freight train bearing down on me, and I could do nothing to stop it. While much has changed considerably for me since then, I do still occasionally struggle with falling asleep. I still sometimes lie awake for hours, wondering if the crickets I am hearing are real or just Mr. T pretending to be a cricket.

The insomnia is brutal. I tried to take a bypass ramp via alcohol and Nyquil to avoid it, but it turns out that I was just delaying the inevitable, direct route I would have to travel later in order to make real change. There is no shortcut here; you either deal with that shit now, or you deal with it later. For me, everything would soon change for the better, but at the time, I was completely in survival mode.

CHAPTER 3

THE JOURNEY BEGINS

Gift from the Gods
Fall 2016

I had been getting blood work done for several years, even before Mr. T arrived on the scene. I'd go to a private lab for testing and would then analyze the data to see what was off and how my health could be improved. With Mr. T, I was even more interested in my blood work. I was looking for a cause and figured lab tests were as good a place as any to find one.

I was playing Dr. Sean again, but I knew I couldn't tackle the medical side alone. I needed help reviewing my labs, and I wanted to work with someone who would go through the results in detail, discussing them with me in a way I could understand. A friend recommended a doctor in Santa Cruz. I'll call him Dr. X in order to maintain confidentiality.

Santa Cruz was pretty far from where I lived, but I had a couple projects down that way so figured it was worth a trip. I knew that if it was a good fit, I would be able to make it work. When I first contacted the office, I was told that Dr. X was not taking on any new patients. They put me on a waiting list and promised to be in touch. About four months later, the office emailed letting me know there was an opening. Something inside me knew that I needed to do this. I couldn't really afford an out-of-network doctor, but I also couldn't afford to go out of my mind. "Sign me up."

From the moment I met Dr. X, I liked him. I could tell that he really cared, unlike the doctor I'd seen at Kaiser. When I brought up Mr. T, I prepared myself for one of the shots to the heart that I'd become so accustomed to over the last four years, but it never came. Instead, Dr. X told me that he was 100% certain that I could either get rid of my T or conquer it, and I believed him.

Dr. X ordered some blood work, which showed nothing out of the norm. Other than my usual high cholesterol, everything was fine. After a few appointments, he started to help me confront my issues. He told me, "You need to be kinder to yourself and stop holding so much inside."

I knew he was right, but how could I learn to be kinder to myself and to let go of things? To be honest, I thought I could handle the kindness part. It would take some work, but I could get there. But letting go of things? That was a whole different animal. I had no idea how to even start letting go. I had no clue where to look or what to do. "But what if it's the root cause of everything going on?" I thought.

I knew I was being too hard on myself. I was tightly wound and had a bunch of crap buried in my unconscious, and it was boiling over. This, combined with my being hyper-focused on Mr. T, could be causing, or at the very least contributing to, my problems. Forget about what the ear doctor had said about it being all about mid-range hearing loss. Dr. Sean and Dr. X were both calling bullshit on that.

After six months of working with Dr. X, focusing on general health and lifestyle practices (sleep habits, supplementation, nutrition, etc.), he mentioned that I might consider trying some deeper work.

"Deeper work," I said, "that sounds interesting. What do you mean?"

"Well," he replied, "it involves using different types of medicines to put yourself into a state where you can get into your own head and do work on yourself. We call it meditation work or a journey."

"What are the medicines?" I asked.

"Generally, we start with MDMA and then move on to Psilocybin."

"Hmm," I said, "that sounds interesting but also a little scary...actually a lot scary. Let me think about it." So I thought, and thought, and thought. I had only had a couple of prior experiences with each of those substances, and both had been more than 30 years prior. I had taken mushrooms a couple of times in high school, but they hadn't really done anything for me. I suppose the dosage had been too low or they might have been from the local market. A few years after that, I had taken Ecstasy at a rave. I remember it feeling good, but I had no idea how something like that could help me explore my psyche.

And yet, what did I have to lose? Perhaps I would just have to have faith and let go of my fear. Ultimately, I trusted Dr. X, and I knew that this was probably part of his master plan to help me conquer

Mr. T. Quite frankly, I was eager to get my life back, not just from Mr. T, but from whatever else was eating me up inside. The causes of my problems were locked in a private, secure vault in my mind, and Dr. X knew that there was only one way for me to access the buried information.

So we scheduled a time for my first meditation journey. It was about six weeks away, in what would be the early summer of 2017, and I was a little excited and a lot scared. Luckily, I have the best partner in the world. When I told Catlin what the plan was, she just said, "I think it's a great idea. You should do it."

"Man," I thought, "how did I get so lucky?"

A few days before my session, I got sick. I emailed Dr. X and told him that I didn't think I would be able to make it and that I would need to reschedule. He was super accommodating and didn't analyze my resistance.

Truth be told, I was scared and looking for a way out. I was sick, yes, but not that sick. In fact, I had probably just made myself sick in order to get out of the session. And when it came time for the rescheduled session, I was sick again. Dr. X was great about the whole thing; I'm pretty sure this wasn't his first time dealing with a patient getting "sick" before jumping into this kind of treatment. Still, I started to get down on myself. I doubted whether the good doctor would want to waste his time on me. I felt like I was letting everyone down, especially myself.

What if I Just Freeze my Balls Off?

At around the time I was about to take the plunge with Dr. X, we moved into a house with an old pool. It was empty and lined with mud at the bottom, but I was determined to get water in it so that we could have a fun summer of swimming. It turned out great. We used the crap out of that thing. Every day we were home that summer, we were in the pool. Usually, we were in it several times a day. Since the pool wasn't heated, it was at its best on the very hot days, but, most of the time, the adults would find sanctuary on a float, while the kids splashed around, staying warm as kids do. As fall approached, the pool temperature dropped rapidly. I jumped in every morning, keeping up my cold water immersion as distraction from Mr. T. Initially, the pool was around 65 degrees, but quickly it fell to 60, 58, 55. Yikes.

"Wow," I thought, "fuck the four espressos in the morning. Who needs that when you can do this?"

I rarely missed a day. Often, I would dunk morning and evening, and maybe even during lunch if I was around. I made some rules for myself to help me make the plunge. One, don't think. Two, don't delay. Three, just go.

The pool was like a cold shower on steroids, and it did several things for me. First, it changed my state of mind. If I was in a funk, all I had to do was jump in that fucking pool and the funk was gone, just like that. Not gone forever, of course, but jumping in acted like a reboot for my operating system. Much like a cold shower, it made me forget everything that was bothering me for at least 15 minutes. Second, it helped me overcome my hatred of cold water and showed me the power of mind over matter. I discovered that I could get my mind into a state of being ready to make the jump without hesitation. When the days got short and it was still dark at 6:00 AM, I was in that pool. When it was pouring rain, I was in that pool. When I hated the thought of jumping in, I jumped in anyway.

Catlin was a rock star when it came to the pool, too. Over and over, in her own way, she has shown her support of my journey with Mr. T. She has always gone in the pool with me on weekends and when she has the time. I thought she was great when she jumped in when the pool was in the low 60s, but then the 50s hit, and she jumped right in. High 40s? She was in. Mid forties? In, in, in. She tells me it's because she likes it, but I don't buy that. She does it to show her support and love.

For the first couple of months, I would dive into the deep end, swim to the shallow side, and then get the fuck out. But, gradually, I stayed in longer and longer. As I'm writing this, the pool is around 48 degrees. This morning, I stayed in for about a minute. It was like a supercharger for my system--such a great way to start the day. My only concern is that spring and summer are fast approaching. What will I do when the pool gets back into the 60s and 70s?

The pool has helped me immensely. It hasn't frozen my balls off yet, and whenever I have considered taking an antidepressant or reaching for a Valium, the pool has always been there for me and has helped my mental state considerably. In fact, it has never let me down.

A Huge Hole in my Heart

Despite the relief I was getting from the cold water, Mr. T was as bad as ever. I was avoiding my chances to possibly make some real changes with Dr. X, and things seemed to be getting worse in the meantime. The noise had migrated to my left side, and my right side seemed louder than it had been just the year before. To make matters far worse, in August of 2017, my Mom became suddenly and gravely sick and passed away a week later. There wasn't even a chance for us to say our goodbyes. She was sick, and then she was gone. I was devastated. I had the greatest Mom in the world, and we were extremely close. I had no idea how I would ever be able to survive without her. I amped up my routine of drinking every evening and popping pills whenever necessary. Everything seemed to be getting worse, from my T to my emotional state, to my lack of motivation, and, of course, my growing fears. I had to do something. I had to trust Dr. X.

MTB Trip Gone Right

Before I could go back to Dr. X, though, there was one more thing I needed to do. It had been over a year since my disastrous MTB trip to Italy. One day, my friends asked if I'd like to go back. They told me that this trip was going to be different; we were going to go on a hut-to-hut traverse through the Dolomites. Although I had sworn never again to go on another international MTB trip, there was something inside me telling me that I had to go. I needed to show myself that I could handle it. I needed to prove that I wasn't going to surrender without a fight.

There was another reason I felt more comfortable this time around. My friend Steve would be going as well, the same Steve who also suffered from T. This reassured me that I would have support if I needed it. So I signed up.

As the trip drew closer, I wanted to back out. I hadn't been riding enough, and the memories of my last trip haunted me. Plus, just six weeks before the trip was when my mom had died. At that point, my friends realized I was probably not going to go, and they all understood. And yet, a few days before the trip, I still hadn't bailed. My gear was all laid out, my bike was tuned and ready, and I was getting in a few extra rides to prepare.

I told Catlin that I didn't think I could do it.

"Love, just go," she replied. "I know you may not be sure, but it will be good for you to get some space for a few days and hang out with your friends."

Even though Catlin wasn't privy to how bad things had been on the earlier Dolomites trip, I took what she told me and found comfort in her confidence. The morning of my departure, I was still on the fence. But now I could feel something, or someone, pushing me along. It wasn't just Catlin. I think it was also my mom. Taking plenty of deep breaths along the way, I packed my emergency survival kit of Valium, Nyquil, and Melatonin and headed for the San Francisco airport, where I met up with some friends, and off we went.

When we landed in Munich, we were picked up for a 3-hour van ride to our starting point in Italy. It was great having Steve around. Even though we didn't talk about our respective issues with T, I knew he was there if I needed him.

Fortunately, this trip went far better than the last one. Mr. T was still there, but at least he seemed more content on the bike. In fact, I was actually able to enjoy the trip and appreciate the sights, the food, the wine, and my friends, all without the help of a Valium.

The fact that Steve was on the trip was huge for me. It took away a lot of my fear. He was like a parachute, ready to deploy if I needed him. I'd had no such safety net on the previous trip. Of course, my friends on that trip would have helped if they knew I needed it. Heck, one of them was even a doctor. But sympathetic support is nothing like support from someone who has experienced T firsthand. Empathic support is powerful and can transform a terrible trip into a wonderful adventure. I am hopeful that I won't need to have Steve with me next time I travel for a ride. I enjoy his company and would love to have him along, but if Mr. T is still around and it's only T and me, I'm determined to find a way to enjoy the ride just the two of us.

In the end, that trip showed that, while my life with T has sometimes been a living nightmare, it has also revealed an inner strength I didn't know I had. It has sent me on a path of self-discovery, understanding, and acceptance. These realizations began to surface during that second riding trip in Italy, but only loosely and vaguely. They would become much more strongly rooted down the road, through the journey of a lifetime on which I was about to embark. It would be a journey that would change everything.

Journey I
October 2017

The day for my first medicinal journey finally arrived in the fall of 2017. I was super nervous and considered backing out. It was a cold, damp Monday, and I didn't feel like driving the hour and a half to Dr. X's house, but I kept telling myself that I needed to at least get there.

"If it doesn't feel right," I thought, "I don't have to do it."

I hadn't mentioned to Catlin that I was planning on doing it that day, so I called her on my drive down. It may sound odd that I hadn't discussed it with her beforehand, but it shows how certain I was that I wouldn't follow through. I didn't want to tell her it was happening, only to have to tell her that it wasn't.

"Do you really think this is a good time for you to do that?" she asked. "I mean, your mom just died, and you have been a bit of a mess for the last few months." She was right, of course. I had been a mess, but for a lot longer than a few months.

"And what if you have a bad trip?" she asked.

I latched onto this question and began to tailspin. Maybe this wasn't such a good idea. Maybe it would just make things worse. And yet, maybe it was my exit card. I told Catlin I would make my final decision when I arrived.

At around 10:00AM, I knocked on the front door. Dr. X answered. As we exchanged small talk, he led me into an upstairs room of his home overlooking the Monterey Bay. It was very Zen and comfortable. There was a futon in the middle of the room, beautiful art hanging on the walls, much of which was from African countries. We sat and talked for a while.

"How are you feeling?" he asked.

I told him I was nervous and mentioned my conversation with Catlin. "What if I have a bad trip?" I asked.

"There is no such thing as a bad trip," he replied. "You are going to be fine. Just open up and trust the medicine." With his encouragement, I made the decision to stay. The bottom line for me was this: nothing else was working, so what the hell did I have to lose?

Gently, Dr. X gave me the rundown on what would happen: I would be taking MDMA while lying down with my eyes closed. He would play music to help guide me on my journey and would also be there to help if I got stuck or needed to tell him something. Then he left the room to get the medicine. When he returned, we did a sage blessing and he handed me a bowl with a pill in it and a glass of water. I felt like I was in a scene from *The Matrix* or *Alice in Wonderland*. I reached out, picked up the pill, put it in my mouth, and swallowed. Right away, I wanted to turn back, cough it up, pull the rip cord, and head back home. But I kept my cool and tried to keep moving forward. Dr. X explained that it would take about 35 to 45 minutes for the medicine to begin to kick in, so he left the room for a bit while we waited. I did some stretches and tried to relax. When he came back, I was lying back down on the futon and starting to feel something, still very skeptical at this point.

I kept thinking, "How is this party drug going to help me?" But when Dr. X started the music, I felt myself slipping. Soon, I was gone, deep into another world.

As I was lying there, the first thing I noticed was that Mr. T had started to fade away and, soon enough, the noise was gone for the first time in two years. MDMA is not a hallucinogen. Still, I saw a visual image of Mr. T. He appeared as a box, about the size of a pack of cigarettes, with two green worms coming out of both sides, signifying my right and left ears, I believe. We had a conversation.

"Mr. T," I said, "Why are you tormenting me?"

He replied, "Because you're not following your heart."

I listed the various aspects of my life, all the while asking him, "Is this what I am supposed to be following?" But, every time, the answer was no.

Finally, I asked, "Is it you? Are you the key to following my heart?"

"Yes," he replied. I took that to mean that, while I had always been a loving and caring person and had always wanted to help people, my work and my life had gotten in the way. I wasn't fulfilling my heart's desire to help others. Perhaps, I realized, I had been given Mr. T in order to learn about him, find my own way with him, and then share what I've learned to help others.

"Yes, that's it," I thought. "I am unhappy, because I am not following my heart. What I want most is to help others who are also suffering from T."

My journey continued for another four hours, and it was truly incredible. It not only involved Mr. T, but also my mom. I saw our life together and, remembering her passing, I felt like my chest was at once constricted by, and ready to explode with, sadness. Perhaps this was when I first began to let go.

Dr. X kept a close eye on me the whole time, checking in occasionally to make sure that I was doing okay. At one point, he spoke to me, very close to my ear, but it sounded like he was a million miles away. In the end, when I finally opened my eyes, I was shocked to learn that it had been so long. I had survived my first journey. It had been one of the greatest experiences of my life. Had it changed everything? Of course not. Not yet, at least, but it had given me hope and a new perspective. It had also given me a glimpse into myself. For the first time ever, I felt free to calmly review and process information about my own life.

It's hard to put into words, but when I came out of that journey, I knew that I had been changed forever. I realized that there was lots of work ahead of me, but I also realized that Dr. X had saved me. He had saved me not just from Mr. T, but also from the other things that had been holding me back—all of the things I had been repressing or holding on to far too tightly. I was finally and truly ready to be free and become a better person, lover, and friend.

CHAPTER 4

THE DAYS AFTER

Now I Can Change the World!
Or Not.

In the days after my first journey, I was fired up about helping others with T.

"But how should I do it?" I wondered. Should I start a website or a blog? Should I record a podcast? I puzzled over what people might benefit from the most, but soon realized that what others probably needed was the same thing I had needed: someone they could talk to who wouldn't make things more scary. Someone they could call in the middle of the night and who would understand what they were going through. For the first two years I had battled T, I had longed for that kind of positive support, especially in the middle of the night when the demons were at their worst. I decided that providing support would be my starting point. I would build a platform where people suffering from T could talk to people who actually knew what they were going through.

I told my plan to both Catlin and Dr. X. They were supportive, and yet I could sense some hesitation. I didn't let that phase me. I knew I would need help putting together the platform, and I already had the perfect partner in mind: Steve.

After all, he had been the one to give me so much

hope two years earlier. Plus, Steve was super business-savvy, and I knew he could help me assemble my project in short order. Two short weeks after my journey, I called him to pitch the idea. He had no idea what had triggered this in me. At the time, I was still keeping my sacred medicine work to myself.

We went through our usual small talk for a few minutes before I told him the problem I wanted to address and the solution I wanted to offer. I could feel Steve backing away almost immediately. His replies were short and distant: "Yeah," "Okay."

He listened to my whole spiel and then said, "Man, even when you just bring up T, I start to notice mine again."

He told me he had worked out his own methods for dealing with his and then changed the subject completely.

It appeared to me that Steve didn't want to be involved with anything that had to do with T. He had worked so hard to deal with his own version and was worried that talking about it would act as a trigger. I had never even considered this. Of course, I'm not sure if that is really how Steve felt, but that was what I assumed at the time.

Steve's response really affected me. When we got off of the phone, I thought, "Shit, what about me? If Steve doesn't want to be anywhere near T, even to help others, how am I going to do it?" I was still struggling every day and every night. If the best thing I could do was to erase Mr. T from my mind, how would bringing it to the forefront of my own life help me?

I concluded that it wouldn't. Still, I felt compelled to follow my heart to try to help others, anyway.

First, though, I needed to find a personal solution to my own suffering. I realized that I might have to put my plan to help others on the back burner for a bit. Maybe helping myself was the only way I could one day be truly helpful to others.

Desperate Times Call for Desperate Measures

My first plan for helping myself involved another attempt at meditation. I decided I would put my full focus on Mr. T while meditating, instead of trying to ignore him, and see if it made any difference. Maybe I could turn the tables and scare the shit out of Mr. T for once. I would sit in a room in complete silence with my eyes closed, focusing my energy completely on Mr. T. I did this for a few weeks, and while nothing really changed, it did help me lose some of my fear of Mr. T. Instead of running from him, I was facing him head on.

Overall, though, I still felt pretty unstable. I blamed it on Mr. T, but, looking back, I think I was also depressed. I was upset about Mr. T, I was heartbroken over my mom's death, and I was not enjoying my career. On the bright side, I was healthy in every other way and had the greatest partner and kids in the world. But those good things, the things that really mattered, were losing out to the things that either shouldn't matter as much as they did to me or were totally outside of my control. In other words, my scales were off. I had lost my perspective and was spiraling downward.

I was also maxing out the cold pool plunges. I was going in at least three times each day in an effort to stabilize my emotional state. I had also decided to give *Headspace* another try. I switched my listing preference from 'general meditation' to 'depression,' which consisted of thirty 15-minute sections. I only made it through four.

At that point, I felt like I needed more help, so I reached out to Dr. X. It was a dark, wet evening, and I was still at the work studio. Dr. X called back exactly when he said he would. He could sense I was struggling and offered words of wisdom rooted in his own struggles and experiences. I asked him if he thought I should try an antidepressant.

"Are you feeling suicidal?" he asked.

"No," I replied.

"Then," he said, "you probably don't need one."

Still, he offered to prescribe me something in case I felt like I needed it. I picked up the prescription a couple days later. I think he knew all along that I wouldn't take it, but he wanted me to feel like I had a safety net.

The weeks that followed were tough, but I never took the antidepressant. I considered it, but, ultimately, I felt like I needed to face my problems without the use of additional aides. It felt sort of like I was in an airplane flying straight towards the ground, and I wasn't sure I would be able to stop it in time. Frantic, I adopted a more aggressive regimen involving more exercise and more quality time with my kids. I also moved my work life from the the top shelf of my mind to the bottom.

Cut Loose and Dance

Another thing I knew I needed to work on was letting go and cutting loose. That sounds funny–*working* on letting go. So one day, when I was feeling particularly lousy, I decided to dance. It wasn't because I'm a particularly good dancer. In fact, I fucking hate dancing.

"But what if," I thought, "the worst dancer in the world [me] could crank up the music and just let go? What would happen if I decided to express myself and cut loose with no rules, no judgment, and no one around to watch and laugh at me?"

That day, while home for lunch, I turned on some cool tunes and started dancing around, waving my arms, spinning, and grooving. No doubt, I was worse than the worst dancer at a Phish show, but still, I danced and danced. It felt so good to cut loose and not care for once. Part of me worried that Catlin would walk in, see me, and assume that I had lost my mind for real, but the rest of me kept going.

The dancing helped a lot. I was wound up so tightly, and it gave me a chance to unravel just a bit. It took me back to a playful place I had not known for a long time and helped me realize that perhaps dancing could be a powerful tool for me.

Every day, after finishing my lunchtime groove, I would hit the pool and then the shower. It all made me feel so much better. These days, dancing continues to be a part of my routine. I don't do it as much as I would like, but, sometimes, at night, I'll put on some cool, tribal tunes and let loose. I'll dance. I'll stretch. I'll practice some Martial Arts, and then I'll pretend I'm a hunter stalking prey with a spear, some two thousand years ago. My hope is that one day I'll be able to go to the park and just groove, without any concern for what anyone else thinks. That's when I'll know that I've truly let go, or truly lost my mind.

Just Breathe and Then Freeze, Part II

Some time later, I was talking with my friend Tyler in San Diego, the same friend who had so kindly offered me hope and support—with a side dish of fear—in my early days of suffering from T. Tyler had recently gotten really into the Wim Hof Method (WHM). He had done two of the master's courses and completed certification. Not only was he certified, but he was also a true believer in its efficacy.

Tyler is one of those people I'm lucky to have in my life. He cares so much, will do anything to help, always has something positive to say, and is giving, funny, and kind. We have been friends for over 15 years, and I often think he knows me better than I know myself. So when he suggested I give the WHM another try, I trusted his judgment.

"Dude, you have to come down here for a few days, and I'll walk you through it," he encouraged me.

"Okay," I thought, "What do I have to lose?" If Tyler was willing to take time out of his busy schedule to coach me on breathing, I was going to do it. I booked my flight and headed to North County San Diego.

I arrived at Tyler's house on a Friday with a plan to stay five days. The first thing we did was talk for a while about our lives--our families, work life, you name it. Tyler's dad had died just before my mom did, and Tyler's wife Wendy's mom had passed away a year before, so we connected over our grief and offered each other support.

Tyler took me out to a little, outdoor casita he had built with his dad a few years before. It looked like a miniature version of Dr. X's place, and the similarity provided instant comfort. I lay down on the futon in the middle of room. After some coaching, the session started. The music was great, and the coaching was exceptional, but I was finding it very hard to let go and engage. We did about 30 minutes of pretty intense breathing. I felt good afterwards, but I knew I wasn't doing it right. I had no clue about how to breathe, and it was going to be a long road to get to where I needed to be. How could something we do automatically be so difficult? Watching Tyler breathe, I thought, "Wow, how the fuck does he do that?"

But Tyler could see what was in my way. As he would show me over time, it wasn't that I lacked the ability to move air in and out of my lungs. It was that I was holding onto a giant bag of psychological content I'd lugged along with me, and I wasn't letting go of it.

After I had chilled out in my elevated oxygen state for another 10 or 15 minutes, Tyler said, "Okay man, are you ready for the cold tub?"

"Yep," I replied. I knew I could do that part. I had been going in a 55-degree pool every day for the last month. Granted, I was usually only in it for 20 or 30 seconds, but when I was in, I was *all in*, none of that head-above-the-water nonsense.

Tyler led me over to a tiny box that was maybe three feet long, two feet wide, and two feet deep. "Crap," I said, "How am I going to dive into that?"

"You're not. You're going to stand in it and then slowly sit down up to your neck."

"Slowly," I thought. "Fuck that. I want to be in fast."

"How cold is it?" I asked.

"39 degrees," Tyler replied. Yikes.

Tyler asked me to try to stay in for at least a minute if I could. He noted that a lot of his clients panic after about 30 seconds. I got in and eased my way down.

This was true cold, nothing like what I was used to up north in the pool.

"Okay," Tyler instructed, "Now close your eyes, and breathe calmly." I did as he asked, but I was freezing.

After about four minutes, I began to shake. Tyler said, "Okay, it's time to get out."

"You sure?" I asked. "I can go longer."

"Yes, I'm sure."

It took about five hours before I felt warm again. I had never been so cold in my life.

After my third breathing session that weekend, Tyler asked me more questions about Mr. T and how I was doing. I told him about my journey with Dr. X and how it had helped me. While I was talking about it, I started getting emotional. This was a side of me I had never shown to Tyler before. With tears rolling down my face, I said, "I'm so sorry."

"Sorry? Bro, what are you sorry for? This is the real Sean, the one you have to let out more." At that, he got up and gave me a big, warm hug. It was exactly what I needed, and he knew it.

Like he'd been so many times before, Tyler was right. Here I was apologizing for letting go just a tiny bit, apologizing for feeling something and being my true self.

I realized there was a virtual dam of crap built up deep inside my head and heart that needed to be released. And I also knew this was totally related to my T.

I did two more long sessions with Tyler that weekend and learned a great deal, both about breathing and about myself. I left there with a completely different appreciation for the WHM. Most importantly, I could see how I might benefit from it. I decided to take my new skills back home and keep working hard to see what would happen. I practiced the breathing exercises once each day, then two times a day, then three. My family thought I was going nuts, but I was only doing it to see if it could somehow help me manage Mr. T. I was hopeful that the commitment to breathing and cold-water immersion could make a difference. I didn't know for sure, but I was willing to try anything.

The Dial

After a few weeks of diligently keeping up my breathing exercises, I noticed that the intensity of my T had lowered substantially, especially on my left side. I wondered if the result could actually be real or if it was just me creating things in my mind. It sure seemed real, though. I was a master at monitoring Mr. T's levels. I would check him before and after breathing and, sure enough, there was a big difference. Of course, Mr. T would slowly ramp back up over time, but he was never quite as bad as he had been before.

Despite the progress, I was still having trouble sleeping. Often, I would wake up in the middle of the night to find Mr. T raging over something. I wondered if I could use my new breathing tool in the middle of the night instead of reaching for a Valium. Luckily, the answer was yes. I found that doing some deep breathing for 15-20 minutes would bring down the intensity of Mr. T just enough for me to be able to go back to sleep.

I was pretty excited about this breakthrough. Finally, I had regained some control. It wasn't as much control as I would have wanted, since I hadn't truly learned how to let go, but it was *something*, and that meant a lot. While I didn't believe that a breathing technique was the long-term, stand-alone solution for my problems, I felt it had its place and was happy to be on a positive path.

I kept thinking in my mind: "Thank you Tyler, and thank you, Wim Hof."

CHAPTER 5

THE SECOND JOURNEY

Journey II

A couple of months had passed since my first journey, and it was time to go back in and do some more deep work. This time around, I was more excited than scared. My intentions going in were not so much to explore Mr. T, but rather to look at my childhood and try to uncover other buried issues that might be manifesting in my symptoms.

I showed up at Dr. X's house on a Friday ready to turn the knobs on my unconscious and make some changes. Despite my enthusiasm, I didn't want to go in as deep as I had the first time. I wanted to stay closer to the surface, since I thought that I'd be more effective there, more in control. Looking back, I know this was a mistake.

Dr. X and I went through our routine, and then he handed me the little white pill. This time, I felt no fear. I was ready, I had my tool belt on, and I was going to fix some shit.

Just like last time, when I started to feel the effects of the medicine, Mr. T began fading away. He was gone for the second time in two years, and bam! I was in and ready to get to work.

As it turned out, instead of reviewing my childhood like I had planned, my journey took me back to

Mr. T. I started running through the series of events that had occurred from the moment I first noticed Mr. T until the present.

Summary of Events Since I Had Noticed Mr. T:

1. See commercial on TV about T
2. Go on camping trip and first notice T
3. Research T online
4. Schedule an appointment with the doctor
5. Have a breakdown at a friend's house
6. Can't sleep, so go back to the doctor
7. Talk to Steve about T and learn he has it, too
8. Talk to friend at the gym about T
9. Do more web research
10. Worry that it will get worse and move to my left side
11. Try acupuncture for a few months
12. See an ear specialist
13. Visit Tyler and tell him I have T
14. See another ear specialist
15. Can't sleep and can't focus; T is getting louder
16. Try Craniosacral therapy
17. Try upper cervical chiropractic work
18. Go to see a TMJ specialist

I relived each of these events again and again and again during that journey. It felt like I ran through the play-by-play hundreds of times for each one. And the common thread among them was fear.

I couldn't help but wonder if I'd been set up—if I'd always had that ringing in my ears, but it wasn't until the trigger events happened that I became aware of it.

My conclusion after my second journey was that I had, indeed, been set up...by myself. I'd succumbed to the fear and had lost control of my life. Did I have T? Yes. But that wasn't the question anymore. The real question was: how much of it was now being controlled and influenced by my fears?

Reconsidering The Events
Since I Had Noticed Mr. T:

1. See commercial on TV about T = Fear
2. Go on camping trip and first notice T = Fear
3. Research T online = Fear
4. Schedule an appointment with the doctor = Fear
5. Have a breakdown at friend's house = Fear
6. Can't sleep, so go back to the doctor = Fear
7. Talk to Steve about T and learn he has it, too = Fear
8. Talk to friend at the gym about T = Fear
9. Do more web research = Fear
10. Worry that it will get worse and move to my left side = Fear
11. Try acupuncture for a few months = Fear
12. Go to an ear specialist = Fear
13. Visit Tyler and tell him I have T = Fear
14. Go to another ear specialist = Fear
15. Can't sleep and can't focus; T is getting louder = Fear
16. Try Craniosacral therapy = Fear
17. Try upper cervical chiropractic work = Fear
18. Go to see a TMJ specialist = Fear

"Why was this journey playing out in front of me over and over again?" I wondered. Was I a victim of my own creation? Was my altered state trying to show me what had happened and what role fear had played?

This second journey was different from my first in many ways. While I did end up processing some other content, including stuff about my mom and my work, most of my focus was on my fear and how I could conquer it. But just like in my previous journey, this session unearthed intense emotions in me. I was forced to grapple with some realities about myself and how I was functioning.

I Don't Have Tinnitus…I Don't Have Tinnitus…Wait, I Have Tinnitus

After processing this new information for about a week or so, I concluded that there was something to it, that perhaps fear was the root cause of everything. It seemed reasonable, especially considering my generally hyper-aware mindset.

"But how can I reverse the process?" I wondered. "How can I get rid of all that deep-rooted fear I have buried deep inside of me? If I was responsible for it being there in the first place, certainly I can draw it out, right?"

I knew there would be no quick fix, but it was heartening to feel like I was on the right path. Since I was still completing my breathing exercises two or three times daily, I decided to start incorporating positive thinking into my sessions. I would tell myself that Mr. T was gone, that I no longer had T, or even that I had never had it at all. I would visualize my neural network and the changes that were occurring deep inside, like dials being turned down and adjustments being made to the virtual processor that controlled Mr. T.

I did this for a few weeks, and although I experienced no real changes in T's intensity, my mood improved. Nonetheless, I realized that the work I really needed to accomplish was still located much deeper in my unconscious. I needed to go back and complete what I had intended to do during my second journey. Maybe the message about fear was meant to serve as a map to guide me to the true vault. Maybe my mind was saying, "Look at how this played out. Doesn't it seem compelling? Now explore. It will lead you where you need to go."

So I started exploring.

Just Breathe, Part III

I had been doing the WHM for a couple months when I started feeling like I was stuck. I realized I needed to make another visit to Tyler's breathing/freeze-your-balls-off clinic. Since it was now between Christmas and New Year's, Catlin, our two kids, our dog, and I hit the road for a little winter vacation of relaxing and breathing in San Diego.

Tyler welcomed me and my family with open arms. I told him I was feeling stuck, and after watching me breathe, he agreed that my mechanics could use some serious work. We did three more one-hour sessions of breath work. Tyler coached me through it and provided positive, life-coaching lessons along the way. I could feel my breaths improving—getting smoother and less jerky. I was starting to feel like I could let my thoughts melt away a bit, not a lot yet, but a little. The third day, in particular, was super powerful. We did an hour straight of intense breathing. Afterwards, I felt high. I was soaked with sweat, even though it was cool outside. Once again, I was excited to take my new skills with me back home to see what I might accomplish.

The Shift

With the start of 2018, I was back home and diving into the pool, trying to stay in for over a minute at a time. I was also diving deep into my mind to see if I could find any clues as to what buried content might be manifesting themselves as Mr. T.

"Maybe," I thought, "my fear vault is locked up and guarded so well that I haven't ever been able to release my fears, and so they released themselves in a negative way through Mr. T. Instead, I want to release them in a way that brings me freedom." Dr. Sean was at it again.

When I did my breathing exercises, I would lie on the floor with a mask on my face, a pillow under my head, and earbuds in my ears. Tyler taught me this setup, and I was relieved I could do the work lying down, because I am always uncomfortable sitting with my legs crossed. After a couple weeks of using my new-and-improved WHM skills, my breathing work started shifting. I stopped doing the WHM and started doing focal work instead, reviewing my past, focusing on relationships from my childhood to the present. This part was a secret I kept to myself. Catlin and the kids thought I was just breathing upstairs and had no clue that my M.O. had totally shifted. I had taken on the role of detective. The case? My life.

In general, when I think of meditation, I think of a state where you can clear your mind of everything. I can't even come close to this state, and it's a goal I'd like to accomplish some day. However, I realized while doing my breathing exercises that I could meditate in such a way that my mind would only focus on one thing, rather than the usual hundred or so things over which I'd usually obsess. Progress.

So that is exactly what I started doing and how I was able to focus on my past. I would listen to some sort of Buddhist, bell-type music, do some deep breathing, and then start traveling as deep and far back as possible into my life. I would look for things that had hurt me, scared me, or held me back in some way. Boy, did I find a lot of shit. It made me wonder how I'd made it so far in life.

What I found was a little boy who had often felt scared, had a pretty terrible father, was a massive failure in school, felt like he was regarded as retarded at times, had gotten into drugs at a young age, and had had his heart broken very early on. And that was just the big stuff. It all felt overwhelming.

Strangely, I also felt a little proud. I was proud that I had somehow scraped my way through life and become successful without the help of a solid education or true parenting from my father. I had managed to find and keep a great life partner and had two wonderful kids, and I knew myself to be caring and kind, even though I sometimes needed to work harder on finding ways to express those attributes.

While I now knew where the vault was and at least some of the content, I still had no access to the actual files containing deeper fears, memories, and thought processes. My third journey was quickly approaching, and I knew there was a good chance that I could access the vault then. For the time being, I just kept doing my routine three times a day.

CHAPTER 6

THE THIRD JOURNEY

Pre-Flight

About five days before my next journey into the sacred space, I met with Dr. X near his home to walk on the beach and discuss the upcoming session. I told him about how my breathing had transformed from the WHM into something more meditative, how I had been processing content from my childhood, and how that seemed like a good focus for my next journey. I also explained that I wanted to work on Mr. T by turning a few knobs and moving some levers.

While dealing with Mr. T was still important to me, especially since he was the whole reason I was there, I had come to believe that I could not reason with Mr. T directly. Instead, I had to circumvent him and find someone or something more powerful that could help me deal with him and release the things that were upsetting him, sort of like going to the boss's boss.

I knew that there was a chance that Dr. X was going to move me to Psilocybin for the upcoming journey, since that was the next step in getting into the sacred space. So I asked about it.

"I think you're ready for Psilocybin," he replied. "But what do YOU think?"

I thought I was ready. Up until that point, I had had almost zero experience with mushrooms. As a teenager, I had taken them a couple of times but had never felt anything. I had no real experience and no expectations, but I had immense trust in Dr. X. So if he said I was ready, then I believed I was ready, too.

Of course, I took it all very seriously. There wasn't anything fun about it. My two previous journeys had been very hard work, and I figured this one would be as well. On the Wednesday before my journey, I made sure that all of my work was done. I also set up an email auto-responder to say that I would be out of the office from Thursday until Monday, and I gave my guys Thursday and Friday off, so I wouldn't have anyone or anything to worry about. I didn't drink any alcohol for about a week before the journey. I ate a simple dinner the night before and went to bed early. The next morning, I drank lots of water but consumed nothing else. I hit the pool and then kissed Catlin and the kids goodbye as they went out the door. I was ready. That's when the dreaded migraine hit. I had been getting ocular migraines for about six years or so, every couple of months.

"Fuck," I thought, "Are you kidding me? My journey starts in a couple of hours and I don't even know if I can see well enough to drive there. Get your clothes off, and get your ass back in that pool." I had found that if I jumped in the pool right when I felt a migraine coming on, it would dramatically minimize the migraine's effects. So into the water I went…again. "Okay migraine," I thought, "there is no way you are stopping this from happening." I put my clothes back on and, with my migraine under control, I was ready to go.

A tiny voice inside me kept saying, "Wait, dude, you just have mid-range hearing loss. That's what's causing Mr. T to be so upset. When are you going to learn?"

But I knew there was something else going on, so I ignored that voice and steeled myself to find it.

Journey III—The Trip of a Lifetime
January 2018

It was a rainy Thursday morning when I showed up at Dr. X's house. I was nervous— not eager-to-bail nervous like the first time—but nervous nonetheless. I turned off my cell phone and walked up to the house.

"Good morning," Dr. X greeted me cheerfully at the door. "Are you ready?"

"Yes."

We went upstairs to the same room I had been in twice before, and he explained the day's plan to me. This time, I would be wearing a mask.

"I'm fine with that," I said. "I've spent about an hour and a half in a mask every day for the past three months, so it's not an issue."

"If you need to come out of the mask, that's okay, but try your best to stay in it," he noted. He also provided me with some tips like: Don't try to control your journey; let it take you where you need to go. Also: If it feels like you're off track, just be patient, and you will get back to the place where you need to be.

"If you feel like you're stuck, just let me know," he said. "I'm here to help if you need me."

At that, he headed back downstairs to get the medicine. A few minutes later, he returned with a tray containing a plate of mushrooms, three cocoa beans, and a cup of honey. I thought, "Wow, I don't know much about mushrooms, but that sure looks like a lot." But since I trusted and respected Dr. X, I didn't feel the need to ask further questions. We completed our sage ritual, he instructed me on how to eat the mushrooms and other ingredients, and then he left the room.

My hands were sweaty from nerves, but the prospect of not taking the mushrooms and never finding the solutions to my problems scared me more. I ate until I had finished them all. When Dr. X came back into the room about 20 minutes later, I was lying on the futon but hadn't put the mask on yet.

"How are you feeling?" he asked.

"Good," I replied, "Just starting to feel a little something."

I was still quite skeptical about the effectiveness of the mushrooms and how they would compare to the success I'd already had with MDMA.

Dr. X watched me closely, and it seemed as if he knew exactly when my journey was about to begin, down to the minute. He came over, put the mask on, and told me to enjoy the show. The music started, the curtains came up, and I was in.

It came on very fast and very visually. At first, I held my breath for the moment Mr. T would leave like he had with the two MDMA journeys. But he didn't go.

I also noticed that the music seemed to have lots of coyotes in it, which didn't strike me as bizarre at the time. Suddenly, I was at the bottom of a tube, and there was a fairy spirit guide to my right. She was small and glowing.

"Are you ready?" she asked.

"But what about my T?"

"It seems like you're doing pretty well with him. Let's go. I have lots to show you."

And she did. She took me to places in my mind to which I had previously not been allowed access. Many of them were dark. In fact, we covered all of the major bases: my childhood, my fears, my dad, my mom, my relatives who had passed, school, love, alcohol, my heart, my life, Catlin, my kids, and more. I won't go into all the details. Doing so would be much like when someone tries to tell you about a dream they had; it's hazy and confusing to you, but meaningful and true to them.

Interestingly, the music controlled my journey. It was extremely powerful and would take me to both very dark places and to places that were a little more pleasant. With just a few changes to a note or a shift from a major to minor key, the music could lift me up or push me down. When the music changed, one set was wiped clean and a new set appeared. If I tried to go back to process where I had just been, my fairy spirit guide would say, "Come on. Stop trying to control everything." I tried to obey, to let go, and to trust in the medicine.

There were several moments when I became very emotional. Usually, it was when my mom was involved. While I was okay with having a few tears run out of my mask, I knew I was still holding back. I didn't want to completely lose it in front of Dr. X. Even though I had pretty much left the building, I was holding back out of fear of embarrassment. I did let go, but not as much as I think I could have if I hadn't been so worried. Looking back, I think my ego was still trying to hold on, driving my hesitation.

Of course, Dr. X checked in on me a lot. "Sean," he would say, "how are you? Are you feeling stuck at all? Are you still processing?"

"I'm doing well," I would reply. But, at the same time, I felt paralyzed. I tried to move but found that I couldn't. It wasn't a concern for me at the time, just more of an observation.

At one point, Dr. X left the room for a few minutes. Before he went, he said, "Keep doing the work. Great job. This takes a lot of courage."

I lost track of the time. At one point, when I felt like I had been there for at least eight hours, Dr. X mentioned that I was only two and a half hours in. Then I started trusting the music. I realized that if the music was still playing, there must be plenty of time, and I had to keep doing the work.

Later, Dr. X checked in on me again. "Sean, how are you doing?" he asked.

"Good," I replied.

"You still processing?"

"Yes."

"Okay," he said, "stay in it then. It's only 2:00, so you still have time."

"What?" I thought. "2:00 already? That's what, five hours? Holy crap, I better start getting my shit together." At this point, I felt like a wreck, so I started moving around a bit, still with the mask on.

Dr. X said, "You can take the mask off if you're ready." I took off the mask and opened my eyes for a minute, but it seemed like the room was twice the size it had been when I had come in, so I put the mask right back on.

Slowly, carefully, I took the mask off again. I was ready to be done. I lay on my side for a while and Dr. X asked me, "So how was it?"

"Incredible," I replied, "but I don't know if I could ever do that again." It had been far more intense than I ever imagined.

I added, "It wasn't that much fun."

"Yeah," Dr. X replied, "that didn't look like fun."

Café Gratitude

About a half hour after my journey, Dr. X gave me a little water and asked if I was ready for some food. I was, and, a few minutes later, he returned with a bowl of nuts, dates, oranges, and dark chocolate. It was honestly one of the best presentations I had ever seen, and the the food tasted amazing! After I had finished that plate, he brought out some delicious soup and toast.

I joked with him, saying, "I really only come here for the food." But the truth is that I was deeply touched by his care. We talked a bit about my journey, but I was still pretty fried and had not really processed things yet.

I will be forever grateful to Dr. X. He has been a remarkable doctor, teacher, guide, and friend throughout this entire process. Without him, I certainly would not be in a position to write this book and try to help others suffering from T.

CHAPTER 7

THE THIRD JOURNEY REVIEWED

The Power to Change Everything

My third journey truly changed my life. It opened doors that I had never known existed inside me, but it was by no means a pleasant experience. In fact, it brought up challenging psychological content and gave me a whole lot to process. In many ways, I'm still processing that content to this day.

Hard as it was, and is, it's been a necessary part of my road to recovery, and I feel blessed to have ended up in a set of circumstances that allowed me to pursue this path. I am grateful to Mr. T for leading me to Dr. X, for taking me by the hand or, perhaps more accurately, by the neck and saying, "I will force you to recognize your true problems and to face them—and your true potential—head on. And, in the end, you are going to learn that I am not your problem at all. Instead, I have been your guide."

When I began seeing Dr. X, I thought Mr. T was my problem. Today, I realize that Mr. T was not my problem at all, but rather the means for me to discover the deeper and more insidious problems that had plagued me throughout my life.

Luckily, I have learned from my work that these are problems I can conquer and that I have the power to change anything within me.

Presence

During my journey, when my fairy guide had told me that I seemed to be managing pretty well with Mr. T, my heart had sunk. I had hoped that Mr. T would go away during that journey, just like he had during my previous MDMA ones, but he never did. Instead, he stayed right there with me the entire time. Perhaps this was the first sign that I didn't really need to work to push away Mr. T after all, but, still, I was skeptical and a bit disappointed. My decision to follow the advice Dr. X had given me—to try not to control the journey—allowed me to let go, and away we went.

Several hours into the journey, Mr. T surfaced again. He was bothering me. I was trying to deal with other content, but there was that high-pitched ringing fighting for my attention like an annoying nag insistently tugging at my sleeve. I mentioned it to my guide, and she gently informed me that Mr. T and I were one and the same.

"You have been treating him as a separate entity, as if he were an enemy within yourself," she said, "but you're really one, and there's no need to fight yourself."

Then she explained that I could make him as beautiful or as dark as I wanted him to be. At that, the music took over, and Mr. T dissolved away for the first time.

Ultimately, although all the lessons concerning Mr. T on my journey were very short, they were powerful.

Beyond my fairy spirit guide and Mr. T, the presence of my mother was very much a part of this journey. She was there for sure. At one point, she told me she was with me, and I asked where she was. Within a second or two, Dr. X put his hand on my shoulder. It was as if my mom had reached out and touched me through someone else, and I began to cry. It changed my outlook on everything (and I mean everything) I had previously thought.

Later in my journey, when I was feeling alone and scared, my close relatives who had passed away suddenly appeared all around me, including my mom. They told me that I wasn't alone, that I would never be alone, that they had not abandoned me, and that they were always with me. At this, I shed many tears: tears of joy, tears of sadness, tears of life. Then, just like when I had first encountered my mom, Dr. X placed his hand on my shoulder and head, reassuringly. He and I only had direct contact a few times during my journey. Two of those times were when my mom was with me, and somehow everyone involved knew I needed direct contact with her.

Love

Several other elements from my childhood came up during my third journey, and they were intermingled with who I am today as a person and a father. I will try to write about them in the order in which they played out.

My dad was first. Like most kids, as a young boy, I wanted love from my dad. Unfortunately, I had never found love there, an experience that had nearly broken me. During my journey, I had to confront this reality.

"You have always wanted love from your dad, haven't you?" my spirit guide said.

"Yes," I replied.

"Was there any there?"

"No, none."

"Then," my guide continued, "how is it that you now have so much love to give? How can you, as a man, give your kids so much love when you never experienced it from your father? How can you constantly hug them and tell them how much you love them, when your own father has still never hugged you or told you he loved you? You may be trying to make up for what you never had, but how did you learn what love is to begin with?"

I knew the answer at once. It was because love had come to me in the form of three women. The first was my mom, who had been extremely loving and caring throughout my life. She had been the representation of goodness in our household, and her love for me allowed me to overcome my dad's inability to show affection. She shifted the scales. While my dad's side of the scale was empty of love, her side overflowed.

The second woman was my first true love. We met and fell in love when we were just fourteen, and she changed everything. She was everything I thought I was not; she was beautiful, smart, talented, and loving. My spirit guide told me that she had been given to me as a gift of love. I can only imagine that I was given this gift to help me learn how to love and to make up for the pain and suffering my dad had caused me. I realized during the journey that I had been blaming myself for the failure of my relationship with my first true love for almost thirty years. Enough was enough. Sure, I had made some mistakes, but I was just a kid, and I should have let go of that guilt years before.

The third woman is Catlin. She is my most precious gift, the one that broke the mold. If I were to try to interpret the series of events that led us to one another as anything other than a true gift from the gods, I would be a fool. Catlin is love, pure and simple. Love is part of her core, her DNA. She is love, beauty, wisdom, kindness, and grace.

It is my understanding that these three women transformed me and allowed me to become the person and father I am today. I am deeply grateful Catlin and I can offer to our son and daughter the kind of love they will never question. They can feel it, see it, and take it in every day.

Fear

As my journey continued, my guide and I ventured into the area where some of my most deeply-rooted fears resided, the fears that had formed when I was just a boy. Three in particular stood out.

The first was my fear of a rabid dog that frequented my childhood room at night. I slept in a room with my brother, on the top bed of bunk beds. Often, I would wake up in the middle of the night to discover a terrifying dog on the floor beside our bed, barking and growling at me. I was wide awake and knew it wasn't a dream. I would sit on that top bunk for hours, scared to death. All I wanted to do was to run into my mom's room for comfort, but I was afraid that the dog would get me. Eventually, I would work up the courage and make a break for the door. My mom would calm me down and, eventually, I would fall back asleep. This went on for years.

The second fear arose from a story my father had told me. He grew up in a very small house in East Oakland, CA, a few doors down from where his cousins lived, and it was said that his father, my grandfather, was some sort of medium and could see into people's pasts and futures. Lore has it that, since my dad's cousins' house was haunted, my grandfather was sent to perform an exorcism to free the house from the angry spirits. The spirits had been doing strange things, I was told, like throwing kids across the room in the middle of the night and pinning kids to the ceiling. It had been like scenes from *The Exorcist.*

Although my grandfather had apparently sorted out the situation, hearing about the evil spirits terrified me as a six-year-old boy. I tried to discount them as a bunch of bullshit, but who knows, right? To this day, my dad swears the stories are real. I suppose it would be somewhat inconsistent of me to say that I believed in good spirits, but not the scary kind my dad recalled. If spirits are real, certainly they must all be real.

The third and final fear involved a recurring nightmare I had as a young boy, which, to this day, I cannot quite pin down. The nightmare was so bad that it would end with me vomiting in the bathroom. I think it had something to do with my getting rid of part of my body or soul and then realizing what I had done, later, when it was too late to repair. I still occasionally experience small hints of this nightmare, but I can never recall any details upon waking. It seems that this fear is located deep inside the vault of my unconscious. Through one of my journeys, I hope to one day be able to explore it and be done with it, forever.

So why did my guide lead me to these fears? What lessons did she want me to learn? My understanding is that, although those incidents may not have been real, per se, the fears associated with them are still valid and tangible, no matter who may have tried to invalidate them in my past. Since I had always been told to ignore what scared me, I had locked up my fears in a deep, dark place in my mind where they hadn't belonged and this had wreaked havoc on my inner life.

Through my journey, I also addressed a significant fear I had acquired as an adult: a fear of dying young. I've always been worried that I would get hit with some fatal disease or that something else would happen to me, and I wouldn't be able to live a full life and see my kids and grandkids grow up.

My guide simply said, "Stop worrying; you are not going anywhere for a very long time." And I believed her.

The Real Sean

My fairy spirit guide would try to keep moving me along, so I could see more. On the other hand, my instinct was to push to stay in one place, so I could work on things and make the progress I'd wanted.

At one point, she sighed and said, "Stop trying to control everything. You need to learn that you really have no control."

I started to reply, but she interrupted me, saying, "Always so serious, Sean." She was trying to make me relax, to be less serious, to let things unfold, instead of trying to constantly direct and control my outcome.

This struck a chord with me; I knew she was right.

I was trying to control everything in my life and was always taking things far too seriously. I needed to let go, have fun, and enjoy. So when my guide offered me her hand, I took it and followed her. It was then that the idea of playfulness surfaced.

"I am showing you," my guide said, "the real Sean. For so long, he has camouflaged himself and buried himself in order to protect himself from his fears. But the real Sean needs to be set free."

I noticed that the real Sean was playful and happy. He wasn't as worried or serious as I was, but he was also honest with himself about what he felt. It became a goal for me to "free" this real Sean, the same Sean that Tyler had mentioned seeing when I visited him to work on my breathing.

Drinking

I had been drinking alcohol ever since I was fourteen. My dad was an alcoholic, so it ran in the family. He was never a stumbling drunk, but he was always a heavy, functional drinker. And his drinking seemed to only amplify his negative qualities as a parent.

For the most part, my own drinking had tapered off as I'd aged, but I was still drinking far more than I should have been at the time of my third journey. To be honest, I used to drink really heavily. I used it as a way to escape. I wasn't even sure what I was trying to escape from, but I needed to escape from something, and drinking was my ticket, or at least I was duped into thinking it was.

Long before Mr. T came on the scene, I drank excessively. I had tried to quit a couple of times, but the abstinence never lasted for more than a few days. This had always bothered me, and for many years, I even wondered if I was an alcoholic. During my third journey, when the topic of drinking surfaced, I was surprised.

My spirit guide told me, "Alcohol is lame. I mean, can it do this? Or this?" She showed me elaborate visions I can't even describe looking back.

"Definitely not," I replied. "It can't do any of those things."

We left it at that. And it was enough for me.

Perhaps it's hard to fathom, but I can tell you now that ever since my third journey, my struggle with drinking has naturally melted away, seemingly without effort. The urge to drink just isn't there for me anymore. I've found I don't need it. Perhaps it's because the stresses that were triggering my drinking are gone, or perhaps it's because I have learned how to manage them better. Or, just maybe, it's because I was told and shown by a fairy spirit guide that alcohol is lame, and I'm a quick learner with the right teacher and the right process.

Every so often I still have a drink socially, but the urge to drink in large quantities daily is simply not there. After my journeys, I realized that I wasn't an alcoholic. I had simply developed a really bad habit over the last 30 years, a habit fueled by hidden fears and unexplored psychological content, a habit I was finally ready and able to break.

Are You a Spiritual Person? No...I Mean, Yes

Near the end of my journey, my guide explained to me that life is too short to spend being unhappy and not doing what you love. As I've described, I had been operating out of fear and needed to stop the cycle this had created. I needed to let go of my fears, to let go of my past, to live in the moment, and to trust that things would work out. I also needed to open up my heart to spirituality.

Although I have never been a true believer in religion, my journey changed my perspective to some extent. I was told as a boy that we were Presbyterian, but I had never seen any sign of that in actual practice in our family life. We never went to church, and while I prayed occasionally, I was always pretty uncertain about to whom I was praying or what I thought might happen. I did, however, always feel somewhat spiritual. I felt like we are all a part of something, that the end was not the end, and that our collective journey continued on after death. Even that belief was tenuous for me, though. Perhaps it's more accurate to say that I had always *wanted* to be a believer, but that there had never been enough hard evidence to convince me. My practical side told me that religion and spirituality were far-fetched, but another part of me wanted to believe in the magic of our existence and acknowledge the wonder of what seemed to be proof of a greater force at play.

As it turns out, my grandfather on my mother's side had been a minister, but I never met him. He died long before I was born. My mom was a believer. She wasn't an active participant in the church, but she believed. My dad, on the other hand…well, who really knows. I have never asked him, but I would guess that he doesn't believe in much. When my mom passed away last year, I was angry. My anger made me more of a non-believer for a while. I couldn't understand why such a kind, loving, and giving woman had been taken from me so suddenly when she still had so much life in her and so much love left to give. I certainly did not turn to God in my time of need and grief. Instead, I turned inward. I also relied on Catlin, my kids, my friends, and some family members for support.

But my third journey changed me. It uprooted my previous perspective and opened up a part of my mind to which I'd been closed off. My understanding now is that I've always believed deep-down in something greater, something beyond this life, but I'd always been too frightened to admit my beliefs and too hesitant to embrace them.

I will save you all of the psychedelic details, but I will tell you that I do believe that we continue on to another place after we die. I feel sure that our loved ones who have passed are with us, watching over us and waiting for us to join them in good time. So, am I religious? Maybe. Am I spiritual? Yes, for sure. My journeys helped me embrace that reality.

The Coyote

I will end my investigations into my third journey with this: the first music that had played in that room with Dr. X had included coyotes howling. At the time, I remember thinking, "Oh man, what did I get myself into?" Those were the only true animal sounds I remember from that day, and they were powerful.

After I left Dr. X's house, I decided I wasn't quite ready to re-engage with society yet, so I went for a hike in the foothills. It had been about six hours since taking the mushrooms, so I was pretty sober, but still felt a powerful connection with nature. I hiked slowly in the rain, under the trees, appreciating the sights, sounds, and smells so much more than I ever had before. The trees, the birds, the squirrels, the flowers, the rain and cold…it was all so wonderful. I eventually found my way into the hollow of an old oak tree. I sat there for about an hour, looking up and watching the raindrops getting bigger and bigger as they approached my face.

After I left the tree, I found a small trail and continued my hike. I encountered deer, squirrels, and birds. I was about 200 yards from my car when, suddenly, a beautiful, light-colored coyote came out onto the trail right in front of me. My heart stopped. I wasn't scared, just surprised. He didn't bolt off like other coyotes I had seen in the past. Instead, he looked at me. I said hello to him, and he walked about 50 feet down the trail ahead of me. Then he stopped and pooped right there in the middle of the trail. He kept looking back, as though to make sure I could see what he was doing. Afterwards, he jumped up onto the hillside, very playfully, like he was going after a mouse or gopher, crossed back over the trail, looked at me once more, and headed down the hill. I had never seen a coyote like him before. He was almost white.

When I got back to the car, I thought, "I would really love to see that coyote again." I started driving and had only gone about a quarter of a mile or so when there he was, standing across the road from me.

A few days later, I was listening to the same coyote track that had played at the start of my journey when it hit me: Was the coyote I saw on my hike also my spirit guide? I wasn't sure, but it all seemed a little too perfect to be a mere coincidence. I decided the coyote was my spirit animal, and I told Catlin that I was going to get a tattoo of it over my heart.

"Okay, enough is enough," she replied.

I told her I was only joking. Well, kind of.

"What is happening to me?" I wondered. "Have I lost my fucking mind?"

Given the spirituality, vaults, spirit animals, keys, and fairy spirit guides, it may have seemed to others as if I'd gone completely nuts. But, ironically, I felt saner than I'd ever felt. For the first time in my life, things were starting to make sense.

CHAPTER 8

NOW WHAT?

A New Understanding Between Me and Mr. T

Where was I to go from here? My third journey had been life-changing, like 30 years of intense therapy wrapped into five hours, and the lessons I had learned were invaluable and so spot on. But how was I to apply them in my effort to change my life? The vault had been cracked. I knew I had plenty of work ahead of me, but at least I finally had the keys. I had learned that the real Sean had camouflaged himself years ago as a protective measure, but was now ready to emerge. The real Sean was playful, cocky, loving, fun, and even a little reckless. This was a lot to process and was going to take some time to work through, but I knew it had to be done.

So what were the next steps in my journey? How would I make lemonade out of all these lemons? I decided that, for the time being, I would simply stay on the path by keeping up my breathing, meditation, cold plunges, and healthy eating habits. I also needed to continue with minimal alcohol and caffeine consumption, intermittent fasting, regular exercising, working to be a great father, spending quality time with my family, and not controlling my work schedule so that it didn't rule my life as it had for so many years. Beyond that, I knew I had to trust that I was on the right path. At least I could now identify with clarity some of the major problems, fears, and hang-ups that I would need to address in order to move on more completely.

But, just more than a week after my third journey into the sacred space, I realized I needed to go back in. If you had asked me right after the experience if I was ever going to return, I would have said, "I need some time to think about that." But now I felt a need to go back to work some more things out.

But what about managing Mr. T in the meantime?

Although I had spent very little time on my journey working directly on my issues with Mr. T, I had learned valuable lessons that would help me deal with him moving forward. First, I had learned that I was on the right path and was already doing a good job of managing him. Second, I had learned that Mr. T was a part of me and not a separate entity, as I had previously assumed. We were on the same team, even though it often didn't seem like it. From now on, I decided, we needed to work together. Third, I had learned that Mr. T could be whatever I wanted him to be. Therefore, if I chose to make him into a monster, he would, indeed, be a monster.

Throughout the next few weeks, I began to rethink my relationship with Mr. T in general. I had previously believed that I had been the one trying to fix things by getting rid of him, but maybe it was Mr. T who had been trying to fix me. Maybe Mr. T was looking out for my best interests, after all. Yes, he had tormented me, but maybe that was just to force me to delve into my past and address problems that were impacting my life.

Ultimately, I came to terms with the fact that I might have to live with Mr. T for the rest of my life, but that realization didn't scare me like it used to. It's not that I was ready to concede defeat, but I was at least open to the idea of having him stick around. I also knew that there were a lot of other things I needed to address in order to continue to move forward in my process of letting go.

Fear Factor

The main lesson I had learned from my journey was that I would need to address my fears in order to move forward in my healing and in my life. In the past, I had avoided thinking about fear altogether. But since my journey, I had come to understand that my whole life had been built around all that I had tried to ignore. So I knew that if I had to pick one thing to deal with that would have a positive effect on my life, it would be my fears.

"Maybe," I thought, "it was fear that caused Mr. T to be so upset in the first place."

Perhaps I had become programmed to think that fear was okay and to be in a constant state of fight-or-flight. In fact, I had a few different levels of fear. One consisted of the old, buried fears, the stuff that had scared the shit out of me when I was a young boy, and which my fairy spirit guide had revealed to me. The second included my family and life fears, and the third involved my work and career fears.

Ultimately, when it comes to fear, I have found that the saying, "The only thing to fear is fear itself" rings awfully true. Fear can be helpful if you are trying to decide whether or not a ledge on a trail is too narrow to pass, or whether there's a lion around the corner, but most fears are unfounded; they do us no good, they protect us from nothing, and, at some point, they catch up with us and hold us back. They definitely caught up with me, but, fortunately, I don't think it's too late. Not for me, and not for you.

Whenever I feel worried or fearful about something, I take a moment to reflect and decide whether the cause of my fear is really so scary that it is worth locking up in my fear vault, forever. In fact, when I take a hard look at my life—my days, my hours, and my minutes—and think about all the fears that captured my time and focus, I realize that probably less than one percent of that expenditure had any business being in my vault at all. What an unnecessary collection I had created for no reason.

When it comes down to it, I have a vault filled with thousands upon thousands of unnecessary fears.

In the past, as soon as I consciously decided to associate fear with something, it was as if I were telling myself that it was okay to feel fear the next time the same thought or situation popped up. But now, instead of feeling fear, I can realize when something has no right to be in my vault, and I can let it go.

Fear-Clearing

While I knew I couldn't go back and dig out all of the fears that I had filed away, I tried to crack down on a few of the big ones after my third journey. I also worked to create a new vetting process, so that I could cut out 99.9% of my unfounded fears moving forward. If a thought came up and I associated fear with it, I took a minute to think: "Is there really anything scary here?"

Most often, the answer was no, so I noted that and moved on.

As for those deep, dark fears that had been buried during my childhood and other parts of my life, I was still not sure how to deal with them. I decided to just keep processing what I knew and remembered to hold out hope that at some point, I would get in deeper and cast those fears from my mind forever.

"After all," I thought, "if you can remove your fears, you can conquer anything."

Magic Mushrooms

Before my third journey, I had known very little about Psilocybin. I had listened to podcasts about it once or twice, primarily with Joe Rogan and Tim Ferris. Their discussions about the benefits of mushrooms had made me curious, but not enough to go out and try them on my own. Mostly, I had been skeptical. How could these fungi be so powerful and helpful?

Now I understand. The mushrooms are a portal to

another place, a place with no boundaries or limits and where egos do not reign. Their power to effect positive change leads me to wonder why these gifts from nature are a Schedule 1 restricted substance.

My story could have been very different, particularly if I had stayed with my doctor at Kaiser and had never met Dr. X. More than likely, I would have continued to spiral downwards. The doctors would have told me to go see a psychiatrist, who would have prescribed any number of antidepressants. Perhaps these would have helped me mask my issues, at least for some time, but I don't think they would have helped me solve my problems long-term or helped me get to the root cause of my troubles. My story would likely have ended with me never really being happy again, drinking a lot, and never feeling free from the chains within me.

My understanding is that the Western world has only known about Psilocybin for around 65 to 75 years, which, in the scheme of things, is not very long, so fears abound. The indigenous people of the world, however, have been using it for thousands of years. Perhaps we should trust their wisdom.

All I know is that, for me, Psilocybin opened a door to spirituality and peace for the first time in my life and answered many questions I'd always had. I'm sure there are plenty of people out there who will say that what I saw or learned wasn't real and that it was just an aspect of the psychedelic effect of the medicine.

To those people, I would say, "How do you know that? How can you know if you've never tried it yourself?"

CHAPTER 9

UPDATES

The Calm
January 2018

It had been just over a week since my third journey. I had distanced myself even more from work and spent a great deal of time reviewing my journey and the lessons I had learned. I was also doing my breathing and meditation exercises three times each day.

In the morning, I would start with a 40-minute session using the music from my third journey. It would include some basic breathing, as well as some time spent reflecting on, and reviewing in more detail, the lessons I had learned. It often made me emotional, especially when the music from a particularly intense part of my journey came on, such as when my mom had appeared or I had talked to my deceased family members. I cycled through it all, trying to process what I had learned. First, I would look at the general lesson, and then I would try to study it in more depth.

In the afternoon, I would do my WHM breathing. This would take around 20 to 25 minutes. I tried to keep things on the lighter side during this session by focusing on some mantras I had created and by recalling the more uplifting moments of my journey. I still used the same music, but I was careful to avoid the tracks that might trigger heavy or negative emotions.

Then, at around 8:00 PM, once the kids were asleep in bed, I would do another 40 to 60 minutes of a more detailed review of my experience. I would mix the heavier stuff in with some positive thoughts, such as how lucky I was, and how much I had to be happy about. I would think about Catlin and the kids, about my mom watching over us, about how lucky I was to have found Dr. X, about Tyler's kindness, etc.

A Few of the Mantras From my Sessions:

1. Let go.
2. You have no control.
3. All you have is what is right in front of you, and nothing else.
4. Let the real Sean out—the one who is fun, playful, kind, and giving.
5. Your mom lives on.
6. You are love.
7. Follow your heart.
8. Be happy for others.
9. Mr. T is not your enemy; he is a part of you. He can be as beautiful as you allow him to be.
10. Don't let the demons win or steal any more time from you.

Throughout that week, I felt much calmer as I spent time in my sessions and with these mantras. It may have been due to the journey, itself, or a result of the internal work I had been doing. Maybe it was both. Regardless, Mr. T was also calmer, maybe preoccupied or just relaxing. In fact, I enjoyed a couple of my lightest mornings ever with Mr. T; he was almost completely gone from my right side, which was the side where all of this had started. He also seemed to be resting better and hadn't woken me up at all in the week since my journey. I had not taken a Valium in over two weeks and had not had a drink in ten days. Small victories.

Work was falling by the wayside a bit, but I remained calm. For the first time in my life, something told me that everything was going to be okay. I didn't need to panic. I didn't need to react or engage in fight-or-flight all the time. I just needed to let go and let things unfold.

That was also the week when I started writing this book. I think it was the first time I could think about writing about Mr. T without having to worry that I would make my own condition worse. I didn't plan to write a book. I just started writing and have been writing every day since.

One day, a family situation interrupted my writing. Catlin came into the kitchen with our iPad Pro, showing me a shattered screen.

She said, "Don't get mad, but we had a little accident."

I calmly asked her what had happened. She told me that our son had dropped it in the bathroom and that he was upset and "terrified."

I actually don't care much about material items, but before my journeys, this incident would have ruffled my feathers and gotten me a little heated. It didn't anymore. It didn't even phase me. My only concern was for my son and making sure he knew that it was all okay, that accidents happen, and that the iPad could be fixed. He needed to know that he didn't have to worry. I knew that iPads are replaceable. Damage done to a father-son relationship via anger is not.

In the afternoon of that same day, I discovered that $2,500 in cash I had been meaning to put in the bank was missing from my backpack. I had seen it in there the day before, and, after a little searching around, I realized it must have fallen out. My reaction, and I'm serious here, was, "I hope that the life of the person who found that money is improved because of it."

I actually paused to check myself. What had I just said to myself? On second thought, though, I agreed and repeated, "I hope they have an improved life because of it." Seriously?! What was happening to me?

Easier Said Than Done
January 2018

Although I was doing better with keeping perspective and staying calm, I still really had no idea how to let go. I worked on it daily, which I realize seems like an oxymoron in retrospect, and it's been a struggle for me all along. During my third journey, I had been told that this was one of the biggest lessons I would have to learn: I would need to let go and stop trying to control everything. Deep down, I had known that for a long time, but I had always been unsure about how to do it. While I had been improving in my ability to not sweat the small stuff, that was not really the same thing as letting go of the big stuff. In my mind, fully letting go meant that something would be gone forever.

But how could I let go? What did that even mean?

My only solution was to try to shake off and scare away the thoughts that didn't belong in my head as soon as I had them. I wasn't convinced that this was a long-term solution, though. What if the thoughts kept coming back? It felt to me like the only way I could really let go of unwanted psychological content forever would be to deal with it while I was on a journey. I needed to get deep into my unconscious, really see what was going on, and then release that stuff forever. Some people do this in long-term psychotherapy. For me, it seemed that the journeys could do the trick.

At the same time, though, as part of my tendency to overthink things, I also wondered if the journey version of letting go was circumscribed around a past memory or a thought, as opposed to letting go in general. Perhaps it was just a small part of letting go. Perhaps, in order to really let go, I needed to enter into a constant state of release. That way, I would not only be doing away with old issues, but I also would not be collecting new ones. I felt like a super strong magnet, with all my problems, issues, negative thoughts, and past memories acting like steel. As they came up, I attracted them, and they stuck forever. I needed to lose my magnetic field. That way, the threatening content could just float by me, and what was already stuck to me could release back into space.

But how could I go about demagnetizing myself to negative thoughts, memories, and emotions? I decided that my first step was to become more self-aware. I needed to stop being so casual about what I took in, and I needed to take notice of everything that was trying to stick to me, so that I could actively deflect and protect myself. Up to that point, my lack of aware-ness had created a graveyard full of shit that had set up shop in me.

Consider the Following
January 2018

By this point, it had been two weeks since my third journey, and my program had stayed pretty consistent.

I would do an early morning meditation session, during which I reviewed the things I had learned and the things I was still working on. Then, I would try to find a blank space in my head, the place where noth-ing exists. It was hard to do, especially in the morning, but I got better at it the more I tried. I knew the space existed because I had seen it, if only for a few seconds. My quest was to find that again.

Usually my morning session went something like what follows.

My Morning Session:
1. Drink a light cup of tea, easy on the caffeine.
2. Lie down on the floor with a pillow under my head, earbuds in, and mask on.
3. Turn on the music.
4. Take 5-10 deep breaths.

5. Start the work by asking myself some basic
    questions:
    - *Where are you? On the floor.*
    - *Do you need to be anywhere else?* No.

6. Inevitably, let thoughts of work pop into my head
and then allow my mind to wander.

7. Brush those thoughts aside and tell myself I'll deal
with them later.

8. Consider the following:
    - *What do you have to be thankful for?* Everything.
    - *How blessed are you?* Very.

9. Review my third journey from beginning to end,
    focusing on the major lessons.
    - *How is your T?* I seem to be doing fine with it.
    - *Is it true you wanted love from your dad and
      never received it?* Yes.
    - *Were the fears you had as a boy real? Can you
      let go of them?* Yes and yes.
    - *Can you let go of those fears now?* Yes.
    - *Does your mom live on?* Yes, she lives on in
      spirit through me and my kids.
    - *Who gave you the gift of love and taught you
      what love is?* My mom.
    - *Who was brought to you as a gift to show you
      true love?* Catlin.
    - *What should you do with your love?* Pass it on
      to my kids and Catlin every day.
    - *Where are your family members who have
      passed on?* Still with me.
    - *What do you think about alcohol?*
      It's pretty lame.

- *Is it true you need to stop trying to control everything?* Yes.
- *Is is true there is a playful side to you that needs to be let out?* Yes.
- *Where has this side been?* It's been inside me, hiding, all along.
- *How do you view your T now?* I know it can be as beautiful as I make it.

Melting Away
February 2018

Two to three weeks after I embarked on my third journey, I started noticing a significant change, particularly with regard to Mr. T. I had consistently maintained my program and had been walking the path to self-awareness at a steady pace. I still had not felt the need to take Valium. I also was doing my meditation work two to three times a day, although I had cut back on the breathing by that point. During my sessions, I would try to process the lessons I had learned and to capture that elusive blank space in my head.

Mr. T. and I had also been getting along better. At times, he even seemed to be melting away. I wasn't sure what to make of it, exactly, but I knew it was good news.

"Perhaps," I thought, "it's because of all the work I have done, all the lessons I've learned, and all the time I have spent learning to accept Mr. T while writing this book."

At the same time, I realized it could be that the

deeper work I had done had released years of stress, anxiety, and who knows what else, and that this had quieted Mr. T as well. What I knew for sure was that if I hadn't done the work and gone on the journeys, I would still be popping Valiums and drinking red wine in the middle of the night. I would still be suffering.

The Junkyard
February 2018

After three weeks, I realized that I needed to vary my meditation and breathing work to give these practices a chance to evolve. I backed off a bit on reviewing the lessons I had learned during my third journey. While I still touched on all the key points, I didn't dive as deeply into them as I had been. Meanwhile, although Mr. T was still around, we had reached a sort of tacit under-standing. While I still kept tabs on him occasionally, I wasn't as obsessive about it as I had been before. Even when I thought he might be louder on one side or another, I didn't let it bother me as much. I also hadn't stuck my fingers in my ears to monitor him for over a month. This was a major milestone.

Still, I did feel like I had drifted off course a bit. My scales felt off, and I wondered if I was once again giv-ing too much import to work and other aspects of my functioning that didn't truly matter, at least as far as my psychological health was concerned. At first, I felt discouraged. Where was my progress? But then I real-ized that change doesn't just occur naturally. It requires constant work and attention. Just knowing about something doesn't lead to magical, immediate results.

"Perhaps," I thought, "I have been so focused on the lessons I learned in my journeys that I have dropped the ball on keeping life in perspective and working to enact change in that area. Really, I should have two buckets. In one, I can put the things in my life that really matter: my family, my friends, myself, the beauty of this world, and the joy of helping others. In the second bucket, I can store all the bullshit: my work, events from my past, my financial issues, and all of the other things I hold on to long past the point of productivity."

Don't get me wrong. Some of the things in that second bucket matter, of course. But I was starting to be able to parse out what would matter at the end of my life versus what wouldn't.

I decided I should only focus on the junk bucket when I needed to actively use it, and not when I was trying to meditate, breathe, play with my kids, write, exercise, or cook dinner. I had been trying to change my direction in this way for a long time, but I'd never had such clear intentions before. Now I was going to do everything I could to flip the script. I wouldn't tend to the junk unless I was in the junkyard.

Basically, it all comes down to mindfulness.

"I need to be present in the moment and not constantly somewhere else," I told myself. "If I'm working on the book, I need to be in the book. If I'm cooking dinner, I need to be in the kitchen."

I hadn't been truly living my life in the present moment. Instead, for so much of my life, I had existed somewhere else in my mind, thinking about things that didn't matter in the moment. This needed to change.

Take a Breath
February 2018

I had been taking a break from my breathing program for almost a month, focusing on meditation. It was working well. But after that month, I decided to slowly start reintegrating my breathing work. One reason for this was Hyperhidrosis, a condition from which I have suffered all my life. It makes me sweat excessively, especially under my armpits and especially when I'm nervous. Between my second and third journeys, while doing my breathing work, I had noticed that my sweating had lessened significantly. But lately, it was getting bad again.

"Maybe," I thought, "if I start back up the breathing work, my sweating will mellow out." There were other reasons I wanted to do my breathing exercises, but that was a big motivation for me.

One night, I went to do my meditation work at around 8:00 PM. My mind was wandering, and I could feel the stress in my face and jaw. It was one of the first times I had noticed the physical effects of stress while I was meditating.

It got so bad that I was ready to just stop and watch the Olympics for an hour, but I decided to try breathing for a few minutes instead. I did 12 to 15 deep inhales and exhales, held my breath at the top for a minute or so, and focused on some of the key lessons I had learned. After the second round, I started feeling high. I repeated the same steps maybe eight times or so. The stress was gone, just like that.

As a result, I tweaked my program a bit.

Updated Daily Program:

1. AM SESSION:
   - Take 10 minutes to get centered. Let go of all the crap that doesn't matter.
   - Spend 20 minutes focused on breathing.
   - Complete 4 rounds of 30 to 40 deep breaths, then do a complete exhale and hold it until it's necessary to release. Follow this with a massive inhale. Hold that for a minute or so.
   - Do 2 rounds of 30 very fast breaths followed by a hold at the top.
   - Complete 6-8 rounds of 12-15 super deep breaths with a big hold at the top.
2. LUNCH SESSION:
   - Give *Headspace* another try, this time on the normal setting, not the depression one.
   - Work on letting go.
3. PM SESSION:
   - Spend 10 minutes getting centered.
   - Do 10 minutes of deep breathing. Aim for a big, long hold at the top.
   - Complete 20 to 30 minutes of review work.
   - Ask: Where are you? Who are you? Where are you headed? What will you do there?

Where Am I?
March 2018

Shortly before my fourth journey, I began to ask myself: "I know where I have been over the last three years, but where am I today?"

I had seen major changes take place, especially in the last four months. I was feeling much better mentally and psychologically. Four months prior, I had been on a precipice. On a scale of 1-10, with 10 being the best, I had felt like a 3. Now I felt like a 7 or 8, which was incredible. I had to give myself credit, something I had never really been good at doing, for putting in the work, taking chances, and trying new strategies. I also knew that much of the progress I had made was a direct result of Dr. X and the medicinal journeying we had done.

My breathing, meditation, and cold-water work had helped, but I felt that they were small contributors compared to the medicine. The medicine also worked to bolster my other strategies; the benefits I felt from breathing and meditation were well supported by the journeys. In fact, as I've noted, the journeys allowed me to come into contact with the content that became fodder for my meditation and breathing sessions. The combination of techniques was powerful.

One night, less than a week before my fourth journey, I noticed that Mr. T was quiet, so I decided to do something that I hadn't done in several months; I stuck my fingers in my ears to get a read on him. My right side was very low, and my left side was pretty much gone. This was very big news. It seemed like Mr. T was finally, truly settling down.

There was no doubt that I was experiencing some significant positive changes overall, but I was still struggling quite a bit to engage in my work life. The truth is that I had begun to hate my job. Luckily, since I work for myself, I was able to substantially cut back on my daily hours and the number of jobs I accepted. This was a stressful process, especially because my expenses remained constant, but I felt strongly that I needed to trust and stay the course for a long-term benefit. Something told me that it was okay to be uncertain and that I had to push through my discomfort in order to progress. I was convinced that there were things even with regard to my work life that I had yet to discover.

Meanwhile, I was becoming a better father. I was spending more quality time with my kids, and I had far more patience than I'd had in the past. I spent time and energy taking in their little beings and allowing myself to feel amazed by the two beautiful children Catlin and I had created together. I played with them more, interacted with them more, and contributed more to their daily lives. This was a gift to us all and one with lifelong ramifications.

Another hugely positive change had to do with my drinking. My urge to drink alcohol was gone, and I could go five or six nights in a row without so much as a sip. I attributed this shift to the medicinal work and the vision and conversation I had had with my fairy spirit guide.

Not surprisingly, my sleep had also dramatically improved. I was sleeping through the night and Mr. T seemed to be relaxing comfortably, too.

I had been relying less on pool plunges at this juncture, and yet, one day, with about five days to go before my next journey, I woke up to pouring rain and cold temperatures outside. It must have been in the high 30s, so I knew the pool would be around 45 degrees. I love going in the pool when it's raining, so I grabbed my towel, and off I went! My family watched while getting ready for school and eating breakfast. I marched out the door and, without a moment's hesitation, jumped in the pool. It felt amazing. Here was the big difference: Prior to that day, I would typically go in the pool because I needed to snap out of a funk or escape Mr. T. Now, I was going in simply because I wanted to. It felt great.

One last change during this time was in how I exercised. I had pretty much stopped going to my CrossFit gym, which was totally new and unexpected for me. It wasn't an intentional change; I just slowly stopped showing up. I loved the gym, the workouts, the fitness, and the people, but it had all become a bit of a crutch for me. When I drank too much, I could go to the gym the next day and sweat it out. If I needed to feel better about myself, I could go there to try to outperform my fellow members in workouts and get a rise out of that feeling when I occasionally succeeded. I could go there to get a break from Mr. T, and it would always make me feel better. I could tell people I did CrossFit, and that would make me feel better. My attendance and performance at the gym had been an avenue for me to lift my spirits and support my ego. At the same time, though, the gym had also been a stressful place. CrossFit brought out my strong competitive drive. For me, CrossFit workouts meant 90-100 percent effort, often leaving me rolling on the floor when I was done. Before the workout started, I would be like a racehorse before a race, all revved up waiting for the gate to lift. But I was a sick horse, and I needed a break. I had begun doing some of my workouts at home and later made a plan to get back to mountain biking and to start running trails when the warmer weather arrived. I figured I'd go back to the gym, eventually, but I stepped back to slow things down for a while.

CHAPTER 10

THE FOURTH JOURNEY AND CONCLUSIONS

Pre-Flight: The Game Plan

A week before my fourth journey, I felt ready. For the first time, I knew it deep within my bones. I was still nervous. After all, none of my journeys had been easy, and the last one had been one of the hardest things I had ever experienced. But what had changed for me was that I was now more scared of not going on a journey than of going. I needed to move along my process of self-discovery. I had done so much work since my third journey. Sometimes I would catch myself wondering if I had done too much. I spent so much time and energy processing lessons I'd learned, reflecting on my life, meditating, breathing, trying to apply new tools, and writing this book. I actually felt proud of myself, perhaps for the first time ever. I felt like I was doing something that might have a positive impact on others in ways my larger journey with T had for me.

While working on my intentions for the fourth journey, I discovered one huge difference from the previous three: Mr. T was no longer on my hit list. Hallelujah. Five months earlier, Mr T was the reason I took my first journey. Now, Mr. T wasn't even on my radar, and it felt like a small miracle. I knew that he would be right there with me on journey number four, but instead of shunning him, I planned on welcoming him along. Or, at the very least, being just fine with his presence.

Another thing that really stood out to me was how I had created this version of myself in order to impress others, to fit in, and to feel better about myself. I thought of this as my ego. I had come to learn that my ego had steered me wrong. It had stopped me from being true to myself and real with others, starting at a very young age. I had always tried to compensate for not being "school smart" and not doing well as a result. I had learned to cover up my true experiences and feelings and opinions in order to be accepted by others. It was, for sure, time to let go of this strategy and learn to be more comfortable in my own skin and with my true self. I wanted to become the Sean I'd discovered during my third journey: the playful Sean, the reckless Sean, the kind and caring and helpful Sean. But in order to do so, I first needed to gain a better understanding of the functions and origins of my ego's protective mechanisms.

I also wanted to look my fear directly in the face. As you know, fear had been a huge part of my life and the manifestation of Mr. T. I wanted to stare down my timidity and tell it that I was no longer afraid and that it couldn't control me anymore. I decided I would kindly thank it for the few times it had actually done me good, and then send it on its way.

I wanted to talk to my young and more playful self. I wanted to get back to him and let him out. I wanted to tell him that it would all be okay, that I was sorry I had hidden him away, and that he could now, finally, come out and play.

Journey IV
March 2018

*"Everybody has a plan
until they get punched in the mouth."*
-MIKE TYSON

Despite all of my clear intentions, my fourth journey was a bit of a disaster. I mean, it wasn't a complete loss, but it was definitely a real kick in the nuts. I had a great plan going in. I was prepared, and I had followed the directions, but things didn't go as planned when I entered the sacred space. My third journey had been very difficult, but it had also been extremely productive. This time, I just felt attacked. It was as if I was being told, "Just because you think you are doing the work and are ready doesn't mean you truly are." The medicine forced me to see the real work I needed to accomplish. It wasn't in my past or in my future. It was now; it involved the 'me' that was here right now.

I arrived at Dr. X's house in the afternoon. I had cleared my work schedule starting with the previous day, so I would be in the right mindset upon my arrival. I had done some easy meditation that morning, I'd jumped in the pool, I'd written in my journal, and I'd fasted from food and caffeine. I felt ready. When I arrived at his place, we discussed my intentions for the journey. I tried to simplify by explaining that I wanted to fully let go of the things that were holding me back, especially my fears, so that I would no longer need to hold on so tightly.

A few weeks before the journey, while sorting through my mom's belongings, I had found a picture of myself as a boy in which I looked happy and at ease. I brought the picture along with me for the journey to see if it could help me access the essence of that boy. Before the journey started, Dr. X placed the photo on a table next to a lit candle. Then we did our blessing, and he presented me with the medicine. He reminded me to ask for help if I needed it and said that if I got stuck, I could reach out to him.

At that point, I was feeling nervous and excited. It wasn't until the medicine started to kick in that I began to feel scared. Trying to shake off my fear, I took a deep breath, closed my eyes, and put on the mask. I was hoping to get whisked away on some kind of magic carpet into the land of my unconscious, but instead felt myself caught on a volatile roller coaster of sorts, with the anticipation, the jolts, the fear. I was cold. My body started to shake, and my jaw trembled.

I remember thinking, "Am I in for four or five hours of this?"

I tried to breathe to calm my system, but it didn't help much. Although I thought about reaching out to Dr. X for help, I wanted to ride out the storm on my own. It was like I was in a fight: a fight with myself and with the medicine. The medicine wanted me to let go, but I was refusing to do so. I was trying to control things, and I was paying the price.

Eventually, the trembling stopped, but the bumpy ride continued. There was no fairy spirit guide to counsel me this time, no tube to travel through, no flow of events. It was simply a messy jumble of thoughts and content.

In hindsight, I understand what went on, and it all related to my deep-seated desire for control. In fact, because of it, I was doing the exact opposite of what I had intended. Rather than letting go, I was holding on like a vise, trying to direct the medicine and where it would take me. On my third journey—my first mushroom journey—I had been open because I went into it thinking the mushrooms wouldn't have much of an impact on me. But this time, I knew what I was getting into, and I was fighting it like hell.

"I want to see my mom," I said. The medicine didn't respond.

Instead, I found myself in a sea of wild lights and colors. It wasn't pleasant. It felt volatile. It was cacophonous. Out of the corner of my eye, I caught sight of a personification of my fear and headed toward it. Although I wasn't afraid, I didn't have much time to engage there, as I was whisked away to another place.

Mr. T was right there with me the whole time. I think he was more freaked out by the journey than I was. At one point, I even had to tell him that it would all be okay.

Although there were moments of powerful emotional work during my fourth journey, it was mostly a rocky ride with me fighting the process almost every step of the way.

My Mom

Soon after I began to relinquish my control, I felt my mom there with me. I could smell her rose perfume. It hung in the air around me. Then I felt a hand on my chest. I was unsure if it was her hand or Dr. X's, but I was curious as to why physical contact would come only when she was with me.

Her hand remained on my chest for a long time. I could feel its force.

"I'm sorry," she said, "I'm sorry that I left you with Mr. T, but you ought to be proud of yourself for conquering him. You did conquer him, Sean. You know that, right?"

She went on to tell me that she was sorry for not protecting me from my dad when I was a kid. I told her that an apology wasn't necessary and that she had done all she could.

Although I had never moved during any of my previous three journeys, when my mother was talking to me, I rolled over on my side into what felt like a fetal position.

Then she said, "It's okay to be sad that I'm gone. You don't need to rush away from your grief and sorrow."

At that, I wept like a little boy. She placed her hand on my head, rubbed it softly like she had done when I was upset as a child, and told me everything was going to be okay.

T Time

Up next was the subject of Mr. T. It's a bit hard to place what transpired, but, in effect, my mind told me that I was in control of what I chose to hear in my head. In other words, I had the power to eliminate Mr. T. Then, for the first time in all of my journeys, my heart came onto the scene.

"Hold on here," said my heart. "I'm in charge of things around here and not you, mind. If I say Mr. T goes, then he goes. Simple as that."

"Ahh, I think I get it," I replied, uttering the first sound I'd ever made during a journey. Then the subject changed again.

Little Sean, Meet Big Sean

As I was starting to come out of the medicine, I asked Dr. X if he could hand me the picture from when I was a boy. I still had the mask on and held the picture in front of my face as I pulled it off, so it would be the first thing I would see without the mask. It was a powerful moment. I asked the boy in the picture why he looked so happy and at ease.

"Because I have everything I have always wanted," he replied.

That struck me. Nine-year-old Sean was telling 49-year-old Sean that he was happy, because he now had a loving family. He had everything he had ever wanted: a loving father and a safe place to live. In a way, it felt like little Sean was becoming my own son in a way. Catlin and I had created what I had always longed for as a child. We had created it for our own children. They felt loved and safe and knew their father loved them. I stared at that picture for a very long time, just taking it all in.

Bonfire of a Lifetime

Although that moment with little Sean was critical, I had actually encountered him earlier in my journey. My son had appeared then, too. Looking at them both, I had remembered all of the things I had wanted to release from my concerns and attempts to control. It was a list of about ten things that I had reviewed many times, starting two weeks prior to my journey. I asked little Sean what I should do with them.

"Burn them in a giant fire, and dance around it," he replied.

Together, little Sean, my son, and I started throwing it all in a giant fire and dancing around it.

"Wait, my daughter isn't here," I realized. Suddenly, she appeared and started dancing around the fire with us.

"And where is Catlin?" She appeared, too. We all danced around the fire, blazing with all the shit I had wanted to let go of: fear, shame, guilt, and bad habits.

"Something is still off," I told myself. "Someone is missing. But who?" I realized it was little Catlin, the young girl who had suffered from the same kind of fucked-up childhood as little Sean, and perhaps even more so. She needed to celebrate, too. We had made it. We had navigated through the swamp that was our crappy childhoods and had come out on the other end. We had everything we had always wanted: love and happiness, a feeling of safety, and a sense of being home. We had accomplished all of this together.

The Biggest Lesson

Ultimately, the biggest lesson of journey four had to do with my inability to let go, a factor which had almost derailed my train when I was first going in. Although the medicine eventually won me over and got me back on track, I had fought hard against it.

I also didn't ask for help. I was so set on toughing it out and figuring everything out on my own that I didn't take the hand that was being offered to me by Dr. X. The same old habits of control and fear were rearing their ugly heads again. When it came down to it, I hadn't called out to him because I had been embarrassed about what he would think of me. This meant that my ego was still in full force, kicking and screaming, holding on for dear life.

Perhaps I had also thought too much about my upcoming journey during the weeks leading up to it. I certainly had spent countless hours running through journey number three, when I should have just accepted the lessons and taken it easy for the few weeks before journey four. I had overworked my mind and rooted my intentions so deeply that I wasn't willing to be flexible about how I approached them.

Thus, the most valuable lesson of journey four was that I needed to figure out how to truly let go. Together with that, I needed to learn how to trust, how to let go of my ego, how to not get embarrassed, and how to ask for help. On my journey, I realized that not only were all of these things true when I was in the sacred space, but they were also true for my day-to-day life. I didn't need to wait until I was on a journey to work on my problems. I ought to be working on them at all times. Every day, I needed to work on letting go and letting the real Sean out. Ultimately, while the sacred space is a great place to learn and uncover issues, the real work needs to happen in ordinary life.

Café Gratitude: The Final Lesson

My fourth journey was shorter than my others had been. Afterwards, as before, Dr. X asked if I was hungry.

"Yes, starving," I replied. I also had a cranking headache. I think it was a result of the furious battle I had waged against the medicine and myself.

He left the room and came back fifteen minutes later with a glorious snack plate of food. It was, by far, the most beautiful arrangement that I had ever seen. I was blown away.

"I need to go out to the car and get my phone so I take a picture of this and show Catlin," I thought, but didn't make a move.

I sat there in silence for several minutes, staring at all the food. There were nuts, fruit, berries, and chocolate. I was starving but also too respectful of the work that had gone into the presentation to eat it. All of a sudden, something clicked. Instead of going to get my phone from the car, I reached for my notepad and pen and started drawing.

"This deserves way more than the click of a phone button," I told myself. I also knew I didn't want to remember it that way.

When Dr. X returned, he found me sketching. He expressed his surprise to see me drawing instead of eating.

When I felt like I had all the details, I set down the pad and pen and very slowly started to eat. Even now, I can remember every single detail of that plate.

In that moment, I learned the importance of taking the time to truly absorb things. The lesson for me was that the next time I saw something amazing, whether it was my kids, my family, a cloud, a tree or anything else, instead of reaching for my phone, I ought to take a real moment to absorb, reflect, engage, be present, and, if there's time, draw it.

Are You My Father?

There's a big part of my story that I've yet to really explore. In fact, I've been struggling to decide whether or not to include it. Since it's important to my narrative on multiple levels, I've decided to bite the bullet and go for it. This part of my story highlights the lasting effects of childhood trauma and also shows the potential healing power of medicine work. This branch of my story has been a significant part of my journey over the past year and a half and has impacted me, my T, and my depression and healing; it would feel disingenuous not to include it.

You may remember that, during my first mushroom journey, the topic of my father surfaced. I was asked if I'd ever received love from my father, and I'd answered, "There was never any love there. None at all."

Like many people, I've long been curious about my genetic background. I'd always been told that my great-grandmother on my father's side was 100% Native American. Since my dad has dark skin, this made some sense. But comparing my dad's features with those of his brothers and sisters, I had always thought that he seemed more African American than Native American. I was never concerned; it was just an observation I'd made.

Four years ago, Catlin gave me a DNA test for my birthday. It seemed like a fun thing to do. Catlin asked me what I anticipated the results would be.   I replied, "I don't think there will be any American Indian listed in the results, but there will be a bit of African." When the results came in, Catlin and I poured ourselves some wine and opened them.

100% English/Irish.

This was unexpected. I shared the results with my mom, who was still alive at the time, as she was curious what they had revealed. I asked her about the lack of American Indian blood, a question she handled with an indirect answer:

"That's just a story your dad has always told everyone," she said. "There's no need to mention it to him. Why discredit his story after all these years?"

Some time after my mother had passed away and I'd experienced my first mushroom journey, I spent a day sorting through old photos at my parents' house. I came across an old black-and-white picture of two African American men sitting together on a porch. It must have been taken in Oakland, CA, since that's where my dad grew up. I took a photo of it with my phone, so that I could ask my dad about it when I saw him next. I didn't let myself question it too much, and consciously I assumed it was just a photo of some neighbors or friends.

A month later, my dad came over to our house for a visit, and I showed him the picture. "Hey Dad, who are these guys?" I asked as casually as I could manage.

"Well," he replied. "That's my dad on the right."

I kept quiet, but inside I was exploding. *Something is really off here,* I thought. *There is no way the man in that photo is 100% English/Irish.*

I showed the picture to my two older sisters and brother, too. We realized that we had never seen a photograph of our grandfather before. "How crazy is that?" we asked ourselves.

I became a man obsessed. Something wasn't right, and I was determined to figure out what it was. I ordered both DNA and paternity tests for my dad. I wasn't going to tell him that he was taking the paternity test; I figured I could just sneak it in with the DNA part. Of course, I didn't really need to have him complete both. I could have figured out the truth from the DNA test alone, but I was feeling very impatient, and the paternity test outcomes were promised much sooner than the DNA results. One thing I didn't account for was my dad's refusal to complete the DNA testing.

"You guys don't want to know about my side of the family," he told me and Catlin. We tried to convince him that we did want to know and that this would be helpful in many ways, but he held strong. He's always been stubborn. We were at a loss as to what to do.

A few months later, on a Sunday morning, the day of our wedding anniversary, Catlin and I received a call as we were on our way out the door.

"I'm sorry, but your dad has had a stroke," the voice on the other end told us. "He's being taken to the hospital right now."

Before we rushed out the door, I asked Catlin, "Where are those test materials? If he is going to die, I need to have those tests done first!"

When we arrived at the hospital, we discovered that my dad was in a stable condition. The stroke had been mild, and he was doing pretty well. After a few hours, when things had settled down and visitors had come and gone, I asked him again about taking the the test.

"I have that DNA test," I told him. "I'd really like for you to take it, Dad. Just so I can know more about you and your family." To my surprise, he agreed. I swabbed him for the DNA and paternity tests and sent the samples off the next day. It took a few weeks for the paternity results to arrive by email, where they sat, unviewed, for a few days.

"Just open it," Catlin told me. "He's your dad." She listed all of the features and reasons that made her believe he was my biological father.

"I don't know, love," I replied. "I've never felt like he was my dad."

With some trepidation, we opened the email and read the results: Potential for Paternity: 0%.

I felt lost and ungrounded. It was as though half of everything I had always known and taken for granted had been wiped out in an instant, and there was nothing there to replace it. At first, I felt sad, but gradually I began to feel relieved by a sense of validation. *Fuck, I knew it. I always knew it.*

Over the years, I had watched my dad and wondered how we could be related. It wasn't because of his looks so much as the way he acted, the way he treated other people, and the way he just WAS. *How can this man be my father?* I had always wondered. Now I knew the truth.

The Hunt

I immediately went on a sort of quest to figure out the identity of my biological father. I had no leads. I couldn't wrap my brain around my mother having an affair or another lover, and if you'd known her, you wouldn't be able to, either. She was the last person in the world

I could have ever imagined with an extramarital lover. This is probably why I'd never allowed the thought to consciously cross my mind. I did some digging, hoping to find a journal, a note, a photo—anything really—but I found nothing. I sought out anyone who might hold a clue. My mom still had two living sisters, one of whom was my oldest aunt who had been very close with my mom, so I approached her first. She was shocked. When I told my brothers and sisters, they, too, were blown away.

I tried a few other people but eventually reached what felt like the end of the road with my research. My dad was the last person who might know something. Of course, if this finding was news to him as well, I would be the bearer of what would be a crushing blow to this 85-year-old man in his last years. I asked my siblings and a few close friends to weigh in with opinions about whether or not I should confront my father. The overall consensus was that I shouldn't. Catlin, however, felt I had to. I was torn.

It was now the Spring of 2018. Frustrated, I decided to turn my energy towards preparations for my first group medicine retreat. The second day of the retreat was a mushroom journey. I had gone on a few mushroom journeys already, but this was my first outdoor one, and it turned out to be very powerful. About halfway through my journey, the topic of my childhood surfaced again. The focus was my dad's treatment of me, especially in comparison to how he had treated my brother.

I replayed my memories over and over. I experienced, once again, all of the pain and the hurtful things he had said and done. I remembered the count-less moments I had wondered, *How can this guy be my dad?* And that's when it hit me: *He knew.* He had always known. That's why he'd been such an asshole to me my entire life.

My brother and I shared a room until I was four-teen. It was a very small room, so we had bunk beds. For my brother's birthday that year, he wanted a water-bed, so my dad bought him a king-sized version.

"Where am I going to sleep?" I asked.

"You can sleep on the waterbed with him," my father replied.

I knew this was bullshit. There was no way my brother was going to let that happen. Instead, down came the bunk beds to make room for the waterbed, which took up 80% of the space. For the next two years, I slept on a tiny mattress on the floor, squeezed between the waterbed and the closet. Looking back, I'm shocked my mom allowed it. It made sense that my brother didn't give a shit, and my dad didn't think twice, but I thought my mom might have said something.

During my journey, I replayed that memory and oth-ers like it. The next day, I was out on the back deck of our house pondering what I had learned, seen, and felt. I could feel pressure building in my chest and knew that I needed to talk to my dad.

The next day, I made it happen. I was nervous, but I went into it with all of the courage I could muster, I sat down, and I blurted out everything I knew, after a brief hello.

"Did you know?" I asked him.

"Know what?"

"That you're not my biological father," I replied, and I immediately broke down. My dad claimed that he hadn't known, that he'd suspected something was up with the paternity of my middle brother and sister, but that he'd never suspected it in my case. At the time, I believed him. Later, I began to realize that he was probably not telling me the whole truth. He just didn't want to have to confess that he'd been a part of perpetuating the deception in which I'd been wrapped up for my whole life.

I managed to get a name out of him.

"If you were ever suspicious of anyone, who would that be?"

He mentioned a man with whom my mom used to work, but I didn't give it much thought with regards to my pursuit to find my biological father.

Overall, although the conversation was very hard, it wasn't as bad as I'd imagined it would be. I had gone into it thinking my dad would immediately shut down like I had seen him do so many times before, but he didn't. In fact, I left the house that day feeling closer to him than I ever had before. How's that for irony?

Meanwhile, I suddenly had some very mixed feelings towards my mom. I wanted to be mad at her for keeping the truth from me, but I also figured that she had done it to protect me and to keep the family together. When we had a chance to discuss things, my sisters told me that my mom had always treated me a little differently—a little more special. Looking back now, I see that my mom did tell me the truth, thousands of times, in her own way. She told me through looks, smiles, and hugs as if she were putting down bread crumbs for me to follow. In turn, once I was old enough, I had always protected her from my dad. I'd stood up to him and acted like it was me and her against the world. I suppose, in some ways, it was.

Armed with the little knowledge my dad had provided me, I decided to give Ancestry.com a try. I knew they had a bigger database than what'd I had access to thus far, and I figured it couldn't hurt. When the results came back, the name my dad had mentioned emerged. He was my biological father.

Unfortunately, this man had died back in 2008, but he had a son and a daughter—my brother and sister—who lived fairly close by. For their own reasons, which I respect, they didn't want to have anything to do with me. It was all a bit crushing. My brother had seemed to want to connect at first. We were the same age and had been chatting online and on the phone, we were on track to meet up in person when he pulled the plug on it all. To be honest, I consider it more of their loss than mine, since I am half of someone they were close to whereas they are merely half of someone I never knew. I did find out, however, that my new half brother had gone to the same high school as me. He was a grade below me, but had known a lot of my close friends.

Although I have been unable to connect with my siblings, through the medicine work, I have been able to reconnect with my biological father. I have recalled meeting him once or twice at a very young age and feeling that there was love there. Of course, I wish my mom were still around, so I could ask her all about him. And I wish he were still around, so I could meet him in person. But the medicine work has given me access to them, even though they aren't here, physically.

The medicine work has helped me manage in the face of real setbacks. It has allowed me to handle some significant challenges with more grace and stability than I otherwise could have. Without it, I would have been at a loss.

Tinnitus has brought me both great pain and great gifts. It has revealed things hidden deep within me and helped me discover my truest self. At the moment, I am on my way to becoming a medicine guide. Ultimately, my goal is to help people heal from all sorts of trauma and wounds.

Wu Wei Tea House
January 2019

Almost a year to the date after my first mushroom journey after a six-month break from writing, I found myself back in a place that had come to feel like a second home to me, a place that I hadn't even known about just a year prior: a tea house. A year earlier, in January of 2018, the day after my first mushroom journey, I went to a coffee shop to do some journaling. It was about ten minutes north of where we live, and I chose it because I wasn't worried about running into anyone I knew. I ordered some coffee, sat down, and opened my laptop.

I wrote a few words, but something just didn't feel right. Nagged by the feeling, I got up and left.

There was a tea house near this coffee shop. I'd driven by it several times in the past, but I'd always felt intimidated by it for some reason. I hated tea. Plus, it looked a little too "hippie" for my taste. But, on that rainy afternoon, after a year of passing by, something drew me into that tea shop. It was pretty empty at that time of day, with plenty of seating on pillows, couches, and the floor. People were hanging around with their shoes off. The walls and floor were decorated with exotic artwork and rugs. It had exactly the opposite feel from what I was used to.

I ordered some tea and found a spot. Even though I felt a little uncomfortable, something also felt right. I opened my laptop and started to journal. Before I knew it, two hours had passed. The next day, I found myself back at the tea shop again, writing non-stop for another two hours.

On the third day, the same thing happened. That's when it hit me: was I really just writing thoughts in a journal, or was I writing a book? From that moment on, the tea house became a transformative place for me. While I was there, I could open my mind and hide out from the world. Nobody in my life knew about this magical little spot, and I wasn't telling. I even developed a love of tea.

In time, I connected with other regulars at the tea house. I also developed a friendship with Tracy, the owner, whom I began to view as a sort of wise, welcoming, mystical fairy. The more connected I became, the more I listened. Among other things, I heard people discussing plant medicines, as well as other types of spiritual and healing work. This gave me the confidence to keep writing and open up in ways I had never done before.

Over the past eight months, I've been back in the tea house many times, but not to write. In fact, last spring, a big part of me was finished with my book. But another part, deep inside, wanted me to give it more time; there would be more lessons to share, and I needed to be patient. When I first stopped writing, I was feeling pretty good. I felt like I had finally gotten the upper hand on Mr. T and that the battle was mostly won. I was wrong, of course. There were still many struggles ahead, and I was far from healed.

On the evening of January 15th, as I was writing feverishly and feeling like I was getting close to a solid ending, Tracy came over for a chat. We talked about how I was feeling, my hiatus from writing, and my decision about whether or not to publish. I filled her in about that rainy day a year prior, when I had been drawn into her tea shop for the first time. Tracy listened in her supportive and welcoming way. I even shared with her some of the details of my journeys.

While driving home that night, I had a sudden realization. I had always thought of Tracy as a magical spirit of a woman. Was it possible that she had been my spirit guide on my first mushroom journey? It occurred to me that she fit the image of that fairy in every way.

This all seemed a little too perfect: I had gone on a mushroom journey a year before-- almost to the day--I'd been guided by a fairy spirit, and then the very next day I was pulled into a magical tea shop owned by a fairy spirit woman named Tracy. The tea house was my writing sanctuary, and now, when I needed it most, Tracy had given me the final push to finish my book, asking three questions: "Where are you now? Where are you going? [and] Where have you been?"

Journey 2019

Meanwhile, Dr. X and I set up a journey for early 2019. It was going to be on a Sunday and in the evening and I didn't like the thought of either of those things. All of my other journeys had been on a Monday or a Friday, usually in the morning. I didn't want to have to think and worry about my journey all day long. I just wanted to get in there and get it over with. Nevertheless, I concluded that this was just another one of those things I would need to learn to accept and overcome.

Dr. X and I met a couple days before my journey to talk about the upcoming session and my intentions for it.

"Maybe this time," he said, "you shouldn't try to do any specific work. Instead, you can just relax into it and become one with the earth, people, plants, and love."

From what he said, I knew that Dr. X could sense my reluctance to drop in because of how intense all my other journeys had been. I liked his plan.

For the first time, Mr. T was not on the radar or on my list of things to solve, confront, or tackle.

Dr. X asked me what I wanted in terms of dosage and I told him that I was pretty open to whatever he thought best. To be honest, I felt like it wouldn't matter too much. How much my guard was up would truly decide things.

He suggested that I go for a heroic dose. I wasn't sure what his idea of heroic was, but I agreed.

When I showed up at his house on Sunday afternoon at around 4:00 PM, I was a jittery mess.

"How are you feeling?" he asked me.

"Nervous," I replied.

"Good," he said. "That's just your reverence for the medicine coming through." He then told me that he had decided to drop down the dosage he had originally planned for me, but again I didn't ask what that meant.

I took the medicine at around 5:00 PM. Afterwards, we pulled animal medicine cards as we had often done before. This time, I pulled a new card, the beaver.

After about an hour to an hour and a half, I was lightly in, but not too deep. I had no idea how much I had taken, but I knew that I wouldn't be able to get any deep work done with the present dose.

So when Dr. X checked in on me, I asked for a booster. He obliged, returning with three stems and caps. I ate two and put my mask back on.

Dr. X shifted his music plan, too, when he saw that I wasn't dropping in. It changed from this light, airy arrangement to something much more intense. It felt like it was constantly building, building, building in intensity and force.

I could start to feel the energy in my body building

with the music like nothing I had ever experienced before. I wasn't dropped in or processing, necessarily. Instead, I could simply feel this intense building of energy surging up inside me. My hands started opening and closing in spite of themselves. My breathing intensified and transformed into a growl. As the music continued to escalate, so too did my hand motions and my growling. There was so much energy spreading through me that I had no idea what would come next. I was in uncharted territory. At any moment, I felt like my entire body might explode, but I was strangely okay with it.

After around 5 minutes of this, I sat straight up and let out the most primal yell that has ever come from me. Dr. X was probably ready to make a run for it when he heard it. It was so intense and powerful, my first real release into the space.

I laid back down and it started all over again, the hands, the growling, the explosion of energy…It felt like a massive release of rage, frustration, and energy all at once.

Then something shifted and I was face to face with my T. I was shown that while I had been viewing it as a nightmare, I no longer needed to do that or see it in that way. It was okay; I could open my eyes because the nightmare was over.

Next, I re-experienced my childhood and the ways in which I was made to feel dumb and bad at learning in school. I had always felt at a disadvantage, always been embarrassed, and always tried to figure out how I could just survive. But now my mind revealed to me the very powerful gifts I possessed, gifts which were simply not in line with the norm, especially when it came to elementary school and middle school. So that by the time I hit high school, I had no chance to excel or even survive because I had fallen so far behind. I could no longer catch up or even learn in the way they were teaching, but it wasn't because I was stupid. Instead, it was because my mind worked in a different way. The main lesson from all of this, though, was to forget about all the ways in which I had failed and been failed at school and to move beyond it. I needed to start looking more closely at my mind in the present and using the gifts that I have in order to further develop and thrive with them.

After this lesson, I began a bunch of deep mind filing work. It involved looking back into old files and memories, sorting out what was true from what was untrue, and clearing out the unreal. The work was especially focused on the age range of 13-18 or so. It was intense and deep and allowed me to see the many blurred lines during that time of my life, times that I would continue to have dreams about even some 36 years later. During this session, I began to unblur the lines and clean things up. I am hopeful that by doing so, I released from my life some of the pain, fear, and sorrow I experienced during that time.

By this point, I was in way deeper than I had ever gone before. While most of my other mushroom journeys had felt very visual, this one seemed to be much more cerebral. I wasn't so much viewing images as actually working in my mind on my mind.

I had taken the mask off but kept my eyes closed.

Honestly, it didn't matter either way. The mask had nothing to do with where I was or what I was doing. I also remember reaching out to Dr. X to grasp his hand while I was processing. I was holding on so tightly that I worried I might actually break his hand, but I needed contact with him and I needed support. I couldn't even hear the music anymore, I was so far in.

After all the file work was done, I shifted my focus to my brother and what our childhood together had been like. I had sought out his love over and over again, but he had always seemed to just hate me. I know lots of brothers fight, but this was different. I thought perhaps I had done something wrong or that perhaps I was in some way unworthy of his love. The medicine, however, showed me that the problem had more to do with my brother than it had to do with me. He hated me but it wasn't because of my actions towards him. He had just always harbored this hatred for me and still feels like he does. I could drop the feeling that I was undeserving of his love because there was no love being withheld. There was no love for me at all. In a way, this realization was comforting because it allowed me to finally start to move on.

Then Tinnitus was back on the floor. I was able to separate it from myself and from my mind and to pull it into a separate space of its own. Once we were two entities, I began to attack it with everything I had in me. I had Mr. T up against the ropes and I wasn't going to let up until he dropped. But then, slowly at first, compassion for him began to wash over me. I started to feel badly about the attack I was waging against him.

After all, it was really just an attack on myself. It did no one any good.

Once I began to show Mr. T some compassion, we morphed back into one entity again. I felt whole. Emotions began to wash over me, but all mixed together. I called out for Dr. X.

"I'm here," he said. I sat up and reached out into endless space looking for a hug or an embrace and it came to me. I held on tightly and it felt like I was pulling things back together again. It was the first time I'd ever been able to reach out to Dr. X in that way and I felt like things were starting to open for me. Like I was starting to open myself up to things.

I had learned that T was my teacher rather than my enemy and, like all teachers, he bothered and annoyed me sometimes in order to help me grow. He was a fierce instructor, especially for the first few years, but I was starting to learn my lessons and do my work and so he was beginning to lighten up on me.

I laid back down. I knew it must be super late by this point. After all, I'd been a busy ass beaver chewing through all the issues that had been laid out for me. My gut felt it must be 2:00 AM or so. At one point, I even said to Dr. X, "You can turn the music down. You need to go to bed."

"No," he replied, "It's okay. Just keep doing the work."

I opened my eyes a little while later and saw him moving around with a headlamp on. Later still, I saw him lying between me and the fire and knew it must be late.

When I finally sat up and opened my eyes, Dr. X

was sitting calmly in the corner. Things were still pretty out of whack and I was definitely feeling the medicine.

"What fucking time is it?" I asked.

"I don't know. Do you want me to check?" Dr. X answered coolly and picked up his phone. "It's 7:49."

"7:49 AM?" I was just getting ready to apologize for keeping him up all night when Dr. X replied, "No, PM."

I couldn't believe it. I thought he was making it up so that I would feel better about taking up his whole evening and night. But he showed me his phone and, sure enough, it was 7:49 PM. I had taken the medicine just under three hours before. All of my major work and breakthroughs had happened in the last hour and thirty minutes when the medicine had kicked in. It had felt like it had been days.

In fact, my mushroom journeys usually lasted some-where between 4-6 hours. Usually, I would work and work until everything seemed to be done and then keep working some more. Not this time. I felt closure. I knew I was done and that the work was over for now and I could lie back, relax, and come back to the surface.

Dr. X started to change the music to a much lighter genre. The next song that came on was one of Catlin and my favorites.

"Have you been talking to Cat?" I asked him.

"Maybe," he replied, and, in that moment, I could see her in front of me in all her beauty, all her love, and all her light.

"Sometimes," I said, "Everything we need is right in front of us, isn't it?"

"Yes," he replied. "Yes, it is."

Review of my Story

When I started writing this book, I was hopeful that I could get rid of Mr. T forever. I thought that perhaps if I kept working and trying new things, I could figure out a way to completely eliminate him from my life. I never believed the mid-range hearing loss theory the doctors had spun. I still don't. Over the course of our journey together, I have seen Mr. T rage in anger and I have seen him rest as quietly as a mouse. His quick and capricious cycles have led me to believe he is a reaction to something going on deeper inside of me. To further substantiate that belief, my fears made him worse, my hyper-focus made him worse, and even my obsession with overcoming him made him worse.

And yet, especially at the beginning, I saw Mr. T as the source of all my problems. I was in a deep, dark place and I felt like he was pursuing me out of spite. If you had tried to tell me at the time that Mr. T wasn't my real problem, I never would have believed you.

"No," I would have insisted, "Mr. T is the instigator of it all. He is the one who won't leave me alone. He is the one who holds me hostage with fear. He is the one who keeps me up at night, exacerbates my drinking, forces me to take pills, and makes me want to slip out of my own skin and run away from myself."

I felt so uncomfortable in my body that I wanted to escape from it completely.

Meanwhile, my biggest fear was that my troubles were just beginning. "It's likely," I told myself, "that he will get way worse. He may even eventually drive me mad."

But I wasn't ready to concede. There were too many great things in my life that I wasn't willing to give up. I wanted to improve my condition, and I was determined to find a solution.

Unfortunately, my early attempts at solutions were of no use. They gave me false hope, but no relief. For the most part, they were all external solutions, involving acupuncture, supplements, upper cervical adjustments, and other such things.

It was only when I started working on myself from the inside out that it all began to click. First, there were the breathing exercises and the cold water plunges. Then I added in some meditation. And finally, when I met Dr. X and accepted the help and medicine he offered me, things truly started to change.

But in what way? None of my internal changes really seemed to affect Mr. T, per se. Instead, they helped to change *me*. Slowly, I began to realize that my problem might not be with Mr. T, after all. Perhaps my problem was myself.

I thought back to the beginning of my journey and discovered that when Mr. T had first appeared, I had been totally unprepared mentally to deal with him. As a result, my defenses had been easy to penetrate. I had been overcome with fear while my hope and courage ran in the opposite direction. Mr. T had been a storm, or a Category 5 hurricane, and my little boat had been too weak and poorly built to weather him.

But the tools I was beginning to develop had allowed me to start on the construction of a new boat. This one would be much stronger and built from internal strength, rather than the false hope of external sources. Fear would have no place there.

Mr. T had been a particularly bad storm for me because there had been no way for me to escape. There had been no below-deck area on my boat where I could batten down the hatches and dry off. There had been no breaks from the wind and the pounding rain. At times, it had all been too much for me to handle. But the truth was that I could have been hit by any number of difficulties, and the results would have been the same: I would have let fear overwhelm and almost drown me as all my hope and courage fled.

Today, Mr. T is still right here with me, but he doesn't drive me crazy like he used to…or even phase me, really. Moreover, I can honestly say that Mr. T has changed my life for the better. He forced me to face the storm of my fears and figure out not only how to survive it, but also how to sail through it. Thanks to him, when the next storm hits, I will be better prepared.

The lessons Mr. T taught me were not easy. They were the hardest thing I have ever been through, but they were necessary. I still have a lot of work ahead of me, a lifetime's worth, really, but without Mr. T, I may never have realized what I needed to do until it was too late and until all my enjoyment in life had seeped out of me completely.

In that way, I think Mr. T saved my life. He was a hero I had confused for a villain. Sometimes, I like to think of the ringing in my head as the sound of a new life, symbolizing my ability to find myself, to rediscover my courage, to beat my fears, to reconnect with my lost, younger self and perhaps to access the one thing that my heart had always desired most: an opportunity to help others.

If you are struggling with T, like I was, hang in there. Don't let fear and hopelessness win. Look to your courage and hope as your best knights. Go deep inside yourself, and try to figure out why T was able to break though your defenses in the first place. Make the changes you need to make, even if they are big ones. Take chances and find your own version of Dr. X. Most of all, don't be surprised if you discover at the end of your journey that Mr. T was not actually your problem. It is possible that you'll find that Mr. T was, instead, a crucial part of your solution.

Where I Am Now

For a long time, I let Mr. T become the fall guy for all of my negative feelings. Over time, I've had to learn to acknowledge and accept the reality that there are multiple contributors to my state of mind. I have my mood swings and depressive moments, and the experiences from my past continue to affect me—not to mention the daily interactions with the people in my life.

To this day, I am continuing my work with Dr. X, and it has allowed for healing on multiple levels. In fact, the MDMA journeys are still the only thing that can lift my tinnitus completely. Despite my positive experiences, I have read stories of people who took MDMA and either acquired tinnitus from it or experienced an increase in their existing tinnitus symptoms. Of course, each story has its own variables, but situations like those do make me wonder whether the MDMA was always medical grade, what their state of mind going into the journey was, etc. Still, even in some of my own journeys, especially with mushrooms, I've experienced significant increases in my T. I get terrified when this happens and can't help thinking, "Fuck, did I just go in and make everything worse? Did I screw up some networks instead of repairing them?" Medicine work can be scary. I don't take it lightly, and neither should you if you are considering it. Just know that everyone is different, and while there are risks involved, there can also be great rewards.

I would never argue that anyone needs to do medicine work in order to come to terms with having tinnitus and learning to manage it. Medicine work has absolutely helped me, but others might come to realizations similar to mine through other therapeutic routes. In my mind, the most important component of healing and managing life with tinnitus is recognizing that T is not the enemy. It is not there to drive you crazy or make you lose your mind. It is simply a part of you—it may be a new you or it may be a part of an old you. Regardless, it's just you. And you are strong. You are resilient and you can adjust to, and come to terms with, whatever hand you have been dealt. That's part of what makes us humans so amazing.

Please don't try to resist your T. If I could go back in time and change something, it would probably be how much I resisted for far too long. Instead, try to learn how to bend and sway with your conditions, rather than constantly and aggressively pushing back. I promise that things will go so much better this way. Personally, I have learned to keep in mind that while my T may intensify at times, it will also settle down again. Sometimes, it may even go away completely while I'm on my MDMA journeys. In fact, as I write, I am currently managing my T really well with the help of a very intense mushroom journey I took just a few days ago.

Parting Words

After living and suffering from T for around four years, I can honestly say that I am now better and I feel deep in my bones that my recovery will continue. I still don't know what caused it. I know that T can be caused by a whole litany of problems, which often depend on the individual. I also know that there are millions of people that have it way worse then I do.

And when I say that I am better, I don't mean that Mr. T is gone. In fact, the level is probably about the same today as it was two years ago. In truth, none of my breathing, meditation, or medicine work has done a thing to quiet the noise for more than a few minutes here and there. But what they have done is strengthen my mind. I am better because I am stronger. I have identified and understood my fears. I have looked deeply inside myself and started to let go. I have come back to life with a new passion and appreciation for it.

What I wish for myself, and for you, going forward

is a strong mind and a powerful and prepared outlook. That is what we all need the most. Listen, it's okay to have a ringing in your head. You can be fine with it… You can even be fabulous with it if you learn not to try to battle or solve it, but instead work to love it for what it is.

And yet, I still believe deep down that I can get rid of Mr. T forever. I still believe he is caused by issues buried deep within me. But regardless of what caused him or what might eliminate him, it has been the strengthening of my mind and spirit that have brought me back to life. Moving forward, then, I want to focus on fortifying my mind and becoming a better and more mindful person all around. I hope that you will consider doing the same.

THE END

EPILOGUE

January 2019

A lot has changed since I first started writing this book. Through the course of those changes, and my writing process, I have debated whether or not to follow through with publication. Tinnitus can be a very private experience—often too private. Even today, some five years after I first noticed my own tinnitus, only twenty people in my life know of my battle. I've thus grappled with questions like these: *"Do I really want this to be my story and my legacy? Do I want people to know this much about me? Do I want people to learn that I have T, that I reached the edge and have been majorly fucked up because of it, and that I have done 'medicine' work? How will this affect my family and my kids? Can I handle the criticism, the skeptics, those who will judge my experience? Will publishing make things worse for me?"*

While struggling with these questions, though, the most important question surfaced: *"Would this book have helped me if I'd found it at any point during my own fight with tinnitus?"* The answer to that question was a strong "Yes." So fuck it, I decided. Fuck people knowing everything about me, fuck the critics, fuck the naysayers, fuck them all. If this book helps even one person who is struggling with T—or with some other part of life, for that matter—then publishing it will have been worth it. I hope it can help you.

ACKNOWLEDGMENTS

To Catlin, my partner, my friend, my love. Thank you, love, for all your years of support and unconditional love. You held everything together when it was all falling apart for me. You kept me going and gave me so many reasons to work to overcome my T. When I came home with ideas that even I thought were crazy at the time, like the psychedelic medicine work, instead of questioning me, you gave me your full support. How was I lucky enough to find you? You are truly a gift from the gods. You are the first half of every breath I take, my inhalation.

To Audrey and Wesley, my kids. Although you know nothing now about my experiences with Mr. T, someday you will and I want you to realize what an important part you played in my journey. You were two big reasons for me to keep fighting and searching for a positive solution to my T. When I was really down, all I had to do was look at you and everything felt so much better. Thank you, my two loves.

To Dr. X. This one is hard to put into words. Thank you for giving me hope and showing me the path to healing. You changed my life, all for the better, not just in regards to my T, but when it comes to pretty much everything. You taught me to be kind to myself, to give myself space, to love myself, and to have faith that I could overcome my trials. Your work is invaluable, your caring is infinite, your compassion moves like a gentle breeze, and your wisdom is a river that seems to run forever. You are the gift of a lifetime.

To my Mom. It's still hard to write this without tears streaming down my face. Thank you for teaching me to be a good person. Thank you for the mountains of love you dished out to me so effortlessly. Thank you for finding the courage to have me and carrying that burden alone forever. I miss you so much.

To Tyler. You are the fucking man. You're such a wonderful person, and you helped me find my breath, my rhythm, and my cool. Your positive words and encouragement kept me going through the hardest times. You comforted me by telling me my T would go away, even though you knew it probably wouldn't. Still, you told me that because you love me and you knew it was what I needed to hear. Thank you, brother.

To Steve. Thank you for keeping my lights on when things were dark. Thank you for being such a loving and caring friend. Thank you for telling me it was going to get better. You are a great friend and an exceptional person.

To Dorothy. Thank you from the bottom of my heart. You were my editing angel while writing. I feel so lucky to have found such a skilled editor who could deal with my Wild West writing style. I am by no means a writer, but you helped me bridge the gap by keeping my words intact while, at the same time, ensuring things flowed more smoothly. Thank you for making me feel so comfortable and for being so supportive while helping me turn what was essentially a brain dump into a complete manuscript.

To Allison. Thank you for being such a great sounding board, friend, and editor. When I first went to you with my draft manuscript, I thought you would not want anything to do with it, but instead you were nothing but positive, supportive, and helpful. Thank you!

And, finally, to Mr. T. Thank you for showing up in my life. Without you, I don't know where I would be, but I know for a fact I would not be doing as great as I am today. You took things from me and you almost destroyed me, but that was the admission price of recovery. What you took is dwarfed today by what you gave. Today, I am a better person, husband, partner, father, and friend. You gave me my breath, my mind, and my cool water. You gave me Dr. X, which is to say you gave me a new life. And you gave me the greatest gift of all, something that I have always wanted: the chance to help others. That is exactly what I am going to do. Thank you, Mr. T. I had you all wrong.

For more information,
help, or support, please visit:

www.quietpleasebook.com